The Religion of a Doctor

Religio Medici

by

Sir Thomas Browne

ISBN-13:
978-1718778887

ISBN-10:
1718778880

To the Reader

CERTAINLY that man were greedy of life, who should desire to live when all the world were at an end; and he must needs be very impatient, who would repine at death in the society of all things that suffer under it. Had not almost every man suffered by the press, or were not the tyranny thereof become universal, I had not wanted reason for complaint: but in times wherein I have lived to behold the highest perversion of that excellent invention, the name of his Majesty defamed, the honour of Parliament depraved, the writings of both depravedly, anticipatively, counterfeitly, imprinted: complaints may seem ridiculous in private persons; and men of my condition may be as incapable of affronts, as hopeless of their reparations. And truly had not the duty I owe unto the importunity of friends, and the allegiance I must ever acknowledge unto truth, prevailed with me; the inactivity of my disposition might have made these sufferings continual, and time, that brings other things to light, should have satisfied me in the remedy of its oblivion. But because things evidently false are not only printed, but many things of truth most falsely set forth; in this latter I could not but think myself engaged: for, though we have no power to redress the former, yet in the other reparation being within ourselves, I have at present represented unto the world a full and intended copy of that piece, which was most imperfectly and surreptitiously published before.

This I confess, about seven years past, with some others of affinity thereto, for my private exercise and satisfaction, I had at leisurable hours composed; which being communicated unto one, it became common unto many, and was by transcription successively corrupted, until it arrived in a most depraved copy at the press. He that shall peruse that work, and shall take notice of sundry particulars and personal expressions therein, will easily discern the intention was not publick: and, being a private exercise directed to myself, what is delivered therein was rather a memorial unto me, than an example or rule unto any other: and therefore, if there be any singularity therein correspondent unto the private conceptions of any man, it doth not advantage them; or if dissentaneous thereunto, it no way overthrows them. It was penned in such a place, and with such disadvantage, that (I protest), from the first setting of pen unto paper, I had not the assistance of any good book, whereby to promote my invention, or relieve my memory; and therefore there might be many real lapses therein, which others might take notice of, and more that I suspected myself. It was set down many years past, and was the sense of my conceptions at that time, not an immutable law unto my advancing judgment at all times; and therefore there might be many things therein plausible unto my passed apprehension, which are not agreeable unto my present self. There are many things delivered rhetorically, many expressions therein merely tropical, and as they best illustrate my intention; and therefore also there are many things to be taken in a soft and flexible sense, and not to be called unto the rigid test of reason. Lastly, all that is contained therein is in submission unto maturer discernments; and, as I have declared, shall no further father them than the best and learned judgments shall authorize them: under favour of which considerations, I have made its secrecy publick, and committed the truth thereof to every ingenuous reader.

Thomas Browne.

Part the First

For my religion, though there be several circumstances that might persuade the world I have none at all — as the general scandal of my profession,[1] — the natural course of my studies — the indifferency of my behaviour and discourse in matters of religion (neither violently defending one, nor with that common ardour and contention opposing another) — yet, in despite hereof, I dare without usurpation assume the honourable style of a Christian. Not that I merely owe this title to the font, my education, or the clime wherein I was born, as being bred up either to confirm those principles my parents instilled into my understanding, or by a general consent proceed in the religion of my country; but having, in my riper years and confirmed judgment, seen and examined all, I find myself obliged, by the principles of grace, and the law of mine own reason, to embrace no other name but this. Neither doth herein my zeal so far make me forget the general charity I owe unto humanity, as rather to hate than pity Turks, Infidels, and (what is worse) Jews; rather contenting myself to enjoy that happy style, than maligning those who refuse so glorious a title.

§2. — But, because the name of a Christian is become too general to express our faith — there being a geography of religion as well as lands, and every clime distinguished not only by their laws and limits, but circumscribed by their doctrines and rules of faith — to be particular, I am of that reformed new-cast religion, wherein I dislike nothing but the name; of the same belief our Saviour taught, the apostles disseminated, the fathers authorized, and the martyrs confirmed; but, by the sinister ends of princes, the ambition and avarice of prelates, and the fatal corruption of times, so decayed, impaired, and fallen from its native beauty, that it required the careful and charitable hands of these times to restore it to its primitive integrity. Now, the accidental occasion whereupon, the slender means whereby, the low and abject condition of the person by whom, so good a work was set on foot, which in our adversaries beget contempt and scorn, fills me with wonder, and is the very same objection the insolent pagans first cast at Christ and his disciples.

§3. — Yet have I not so shaken hands with those desperate resolutions who had rather venture at large their decayed bottom, than bring her in to be new-trimmed in the dock — who had rather promiscuously retain all, than abridge any, and obstinately be what they are, than what they have been — as to stand in diameter and sword's point with them. We have reformed from them, not against them: for, omitting those improperations[2] and terms of scurrility betwixt us, which only difference our affections, and not our cause, there is between us one common name and appellation, one faith and necessary body of principles common to us both; and therefore I am not scrupulous to converse and live with them, to enter their churches in defect of ours, and either pray with them or for them. I could never perceive any rational consequences from those many texts which prohibit the children of Israel to pollute themselves with the temples of the heathens; we being all Christians, and not divided by such detested impieties as might profane our prayers, or the place wherein we make them; or that a resolved conscience may not adore her Creator anywhere, especially in places devoted to his service; if their devotions offend him, mine may please him: if theirs profane it, mine may hallow it. Holy water and crucifix (dangerous to the common people) deceive not my judgment, nor abuse my devotion at all. I am, I confess, naturally inclined to that which misguided zeal terms superstition: my common conversation I do acknowledge austere, my behaviour full of rigour, sometimes not without morosity; yet, at my devotion I love to use the civility of my knee, my hat, and hand, with all those outward and sensible motions which may express or promote my invisible devotion. I should violate my own arm rather than a church; nor willingly deface the name of saint or martyr. At the sight of a cross, or crucifix, I can dispense with my hat, but scarce with the thought or memory of my Saviour. I cannot laugh at, but rather pity, the fruitless journeys of pilgrims, or contemn the miserable condition of friars; for, though misplaced in circumstances, there is something in it of * A church-bell, that tolls every day at six and twelve of the clock; at the hearing whereof every one, in what place soever, either of house or street, betakes himself to his prayer, which is commonly directed to the Virgin. devotion. I could never hear the Ave–Mary bell* without an elevation, or think it a sufficient warrant, because they erred in one circumstance, for me to err in all — that is, in silence and dumb contempt. Whilst, therefore, they direct their devotions to her, I offered mine to God; and rectify the errors of their prayers by rightly ordering mine own. At a solemn procession I have wept abundantly, while my consorts, blind with opposition and prejudice, have fallen into an excess of scorn and laughter. There are, questionless, both in Greek, Roman, and African churches, solemnities and ceremonies, whereof the wiser zeals do make a Christian use; and stand condemned by us, not as evil in themselves, but as allurements and baits of superstition to those vulgar heads that look asquint on the face of truth, and those unstable judgments that cannot resist in the narrow point and centre of virtue without a reel or stagger to the circumference.

§4. — As there were many reformers, so likewise many reformations; every country proceeding in a particular way and method, according as their national interest, together with their constitution and clime, inclined them: some angrily and with extremity; others calmly and with mediocrity, not rending, but easily dividing, the community, and leaving an honest possibility of a reconciliation; — which, though peaceable spirits do desire, and may conceive that revolution of time and the mercies of God may effect, yet that judgment that shall consider the present antipathies between the two extremes — their contrarieties in condition, affection, and opinion — may, with the same hopes, expect a union in the poles of heaven.

§5. — But, to difference myself nearer, and draw into a lesser circle; there is no church whose every part so squares unto my conscience, whose articles, constitutions, and customs, seem so consonant unto reason, and, as it were, framed to my particular devotion, as this whereof I hold my belief — the Church of England; to whose faith I am a sworn subject, and therefore, in a double obligation, subscribe unto her articles, and endeavour to observe her constitutions: whatsoever is beyond, as points indifferent, I observe, according to the rules of my private reason, or the humour and fashion of my devotion; neither believing this because Luther affirmed it, nor disproving that because Calvin hath disavouched it. I condemn not all things in the council of Trent, nor approve all in the synod of Dort.[3] In brief, where the Scripture is silent, the church is my text; where that speaks, 'tis but my comment;[4] where there is a joint silence of both, I borrow not the rules of my religion from Rome or Geneva, but from the dictates of my own reason. It is an unjust scandal of our adversaries, and a gross error in ourselves, to compute the nativity of our religion from Henry the Eighth; who, though he rejected the Pope, refused not the faith of Rome,[5] and effected no more than what his own predecessors desired and essayed in ages past, and it was conceived the state of Venice would have attempted in our days.[6] It is as uncharitable a point in us to fall upon those popular scurrilities and opprobrious scoffs of the Bishop of Rome, to whom, as a temporal prince, we owe the duty of good language. I confess there is a cause of passion between us: by his sentence I stand excommunicated; heretic is the best language he affords me: yet can no ear witness I ever returned to him the name of antichrist, man of sin, or whore of Babylon. It is the method of charity to suffer without reaction: those usual satires and invectives of the pulpit may perchance produce a good effect on the vulgar, whose ears are opener to rhetoric than logic; yet do they, in no wise, confirm the faith of wiser believers, who know that a good cause needs not be pardoned by passion, but can sustain itself upon a temperate dispute.

§6. — I could never divide myself from any man upon the difference of an opinion, or be angry with his judgment for not agreeing with me in that from which, perhaps, within a few days, I should dissent myself. I have no genius to disputes in religion: and have often thought it wisdom to decline them, especially upon a disadvantage, or when the cause of truth might suffer in the weakness of my patronage. Where we desire to be informed, 'tis good to contest with men above ourselves; but, to confirm and establish our opinions, 'tis best to argue with judgments below our own, that the frequent spoils and victories over their reasons may settle in ourselves an esteem and confirmed opinion of our own. Every man is not a proper champion for truth, nor fit to take up the gauntlet in the cause of verity; many, from the ignorance of these maxims, and an inconsiderate zeal unto truth, have too rashly charged the troops of error and remain as trophies unto the enemies of truth. A man may be in as just possession of truth as of a city, and yet be forced to surrender; 'tis therefore far better to enjoy her with peace than to hazard her on a battle. If, therefore, there rise any doubts in my way, I do forget them, or at least defer them, till my better settled judgment and more manly reason be able to resolve them; for I perceive every man's own reason is his best OEdipus,⁷ and will, upon a reasonable truce, find a way to loose those bonds wherewith the subtleties of error have enchained our more flexible and tender judgments. In philosophy, where truth seems double-faced, there is no man more paradoxical than myself: but in divinity I love to keep the road; and, though not in an implicit, yet an humble faith, follow the great wheel of the church, by which I move; not reserving any proper poles, or motion from the epicycle of my own brain. By this means I have no gap for heresy, schisms, or errors, of which at present, I hope I shall not injure truth to say, I have no taint or tincture. I must confess my greener studies have been polluted with two or three; not any begotten in the latter centuries, but old and obsolete, such as could never have been revived but by such extravagant and irregular heads as mine. For, indeed, heresies perish not with their authors; but, like the river Arethusa,⁸ though they lose their currents in one place, they rise up again in another. One general council is not able to extirpate one single heresy: it may be cancelled for the present; but revolution of time, and the like aspects from heaven, will restore it, when it will flourish till it be condemned again. For, as though there were metem-psychosis, and the soul of one man passed into another, opinions do find, after certain revolutions, men and minds like those that first begat them. To see ourselves again, we need not look for Plato's * A revolution of certain thousand years, when all things should return unto their former estate, and he be teaching again in his school, as when he delivered this opinion. year:* every man is not only himself; there have been many Diogenes, and as many Timons, though but few of that name; men are lived over again; the world is now as it was in ages past; there was none then, but there hath been some one since, that parallels him, and is, as it were, his revived self.

§7. — Now, the first of mine was that of the Arabians;[2] that the souls of men perished with their bodies, but should yet be raised again at the last day: not that I did absolutely conceive a mortality of the soul, but, if that were (which faith, not philosophy, hath yet thoroughly disproved), and that both entered the grave together, yet I held the same conceit thereof that we all do of the body, that it rise again. Surely it is but the merits of our unworthy natures, if we sleep in darkness until the last alarm. A serious reflex upon my own unworthiness did make me backward from challenging this prerogative of my soul: so that I might enjoy my Saviour at the last, I could with patience be nothing almost unto eternity. The second was that of Origen; that God would not persist in his vengeance for ever, but, after a definite time of his wrath, would release the damned souls from torture; which error I fell into upon a serious contemplation of the great attribute of God, his mercy; and did a little cherish it in myself, because I found therein no malice, and a ready weight to sway me from the other extreme of despair, whereunto melancholy and contemplative natures are too easily disposed. A third there is, which I did never positively maintain or practise, but have often wished it had been consonant to truth, and not offensive to my religion; and that is, the prayer for the dead; whereunto I was inclined from some charitable inducements, whereby I could scarce contain my prayers for a friend at the ringing of a bell, or behold his corpse without an orison for his soul. 'Twas a good way, methought, to be remembered by posterity, and far more noble than a history. These opinions I never maintained with pertinacity, or endeavoured to inveigle any man's belief unto mine, nor so much as ever revealed, or disputed them with my dearest friends; by which means I neither propagated them in others nor confirmed them in myself: but, suffering them to flame upon their own substance, without addition of new fuel, they went out insensibly of themselves; therefore these opinions, though condemned by lawful councils, were not heresies in me, but bare errors, and single lapses of my understanding, without a joint depravity of my will. Those have not only depraved understandings, but diseased affections, which cannot enjoy a singularity without a heresy, or be the author of an opinion without they be of a sect also. This was the villany of the first schism of Lucifer; who was not content to err alone, but drew into his faction many legions; and upon this experience he tempted only Eve, well understanding the communicable nature of sin, and that to deceive but one was tacitly and upon consequence to delude them both.

§8. — That heresies should arise, we have the prophecy of Christ; but, that old ones should be abolished, we hold no prediction. That there must be heresies, is true, not only in our church, but also in any other: even in the doctrines heretical there will be superheresies; and Arians, not only divided from the church, but also among themselves: for heads that are disposed unto schism, and complexionally propense to innovation, are naturally indisposed for a community; nor will be ever confined unto the order or economy of one body; and therefore, when they separate from others, they knit but loosely among themselves; nor contented with a general breach or dichotomy[10] with their church, do subdivide and mince themselves almost into atoms. 'Tis true, that men of singular parts and humours have not been free from singular opinions and conceits in all ages; retaining something, not only beside the opinion of his own church, or any other, but also any particular author; which, notwithstanding, a sober judgment may do without offence or heresy; for there is yet, after all the decrees of councils, and the niceties of the schools, many things, untouched, unimagined, wherein the liberty of an honest reason may play and expatiate with security, and far without the circle of a heresy.

§9. — As for those wingy mysteries in divinity, and airy subtleties in religion, which have unhinged the brains of better heads, they never stretched the *pia mater*[11] of mine. Methinks there be not impossibilities enough in religion for an active faith: the deepest mysteries ours contains have not only been illustrated, but maintained, by syllogism and the rule of reason. I love to lose myself in a mystery; to pursue my reason to an *O altitudo!* 'Tis my solitary recreation to pose my apprehension with those involved enigmas and riddles of the Trinity — with incarnation and resurrection. I can answer all the objections of Satan and my rebellious reason with that odd resolution I learned of Tertullian, "Certum est quia impossibile est." I desire to exercise my faith in the difficultest point; for, to credit ordinary and visible objects, is not faith, but persuasion. Some believe the better for seeing Christ's sepulchre; and, when they have seen the Red Sea, doubt not of the miracle. Now, contrarily, I bless myself, and am thankful, that I lived not in the days of miracles; that I never saw Christ nor his disciples. I would not have been one of those Israelites that passed the Red Sea; nor one of Christ's patients, on whom he wrought his wonders: then had my faith been thrust upon me; nor should I enjoy that greater blessing pronounced to all that believe and saw not. 'Tis an easy and necessary belief, to credit what our eye and sense hath examined. I believe he was dead, and buried, and rose again; and desire to see him in his glory, rather than to contemplate him in his cenotaph or sepulchre. Nor is this much to believe; as we have reason, we owe this faith unto history: they only had the advantage of a bold and noble faith, who lived before his coming, who, upon obscure prophesies and mystical types, could raise a belief, and expect apparent impossibilities.

$10. —'Tis true, there is an edge in all firm belief, and with an easy metaphor we may say, the sword of faith; but in these obscurities I rather use it in the adjunct the apostle gives it, a buckler; under which I conceive a wary combatant may lie invulnerable. Since I was of understanding to know that we knew nothing, my reason hath been more pliable to the will of faith: I am now content to understand a mystery, without a rigid definition, in an easy and Platonic description. That allegorical description * "Sphaera cujus centrum ubique, circumferentia nullibi." of Hermes* pleaseth me beyond all the metaphysical definitions of divines. Where I cannot satisfy my reason, I love to humour my fancy: I had as lieve you tell me that *anima est angelus hominis, est corpus Dei*, as [Greek omitted]; — *lux est umbra Dei*, as *actus perspicui*. Where there is an obscurity too deep for our reason, 'tis good to sit down with a description, periphrasis, or adumbration;[12] for, by acquainting our reason how unable it is to display the visible and obvious effects of nature, it becomes more humble and submissive unto the subtleties of faith: and thus I teach my haggard and unreclaimed reason to stoop unto the lure of faith. I believe there was already a tree, whose fruit our unhappy parents tasted, though, in the same chapter when God forbids it, 'tis positively said, the plants of the field were not yet grown; for God had not caused it to rain upon the earth. I believe that the serpent (if we shall literally understand it), from his proper form and figure, made his motion on his belly, before the curse. I find the trial of the pucelage and virginity of women, which God ordained the Jews, is very fallible. Experience and history informs me that, not only many particular women, but likewise whole nations, have escaped the curse of childbirth, which God seems to pronounce upon the whole sex; yet do I believe that all this is true, which, indeed, my reason would persuade me to be false: and this, I think, is no vulgar part of faith, to believe a thing not only above, but contrary to, reason, and against the arguments of our proper senses.

§11. — In my solitary and retired imagination ("neque enim cum porticus aut me lectulus accepit, desum *mihi*"), I remember I am not alone; and therefore forget not to contemplate him and his attributes, who is ever with me, especially those two mighty ones, his wisdom and eternity. With the one I recreate, with the other I confound, my understanding: for who can speak of eternity without a solecism, or think thereof without an ecstasy? Time we may comprehend; 'tis but five days elder than ourselves, and hath the same horoscope with the world; but, to retire so far back as to apprehend a beginning — to give such an infinite start forwards as to conceive an end — in an essence that we affirm hath neither the one nor the other, it puts my reason to St Paul's sanctuary: my philosophy dares not say the angels can do it. God hath not made a creature that can comprehend him; 'tis a privilege of his own nature: "I am that I am" was his own definition unto Moses; and 'twas a short one to confound mortality, that durst question God, or ask him what he was. Indeed, he only is; all others have and shall be; but, in eternity, there is no distinction of tenses; and therefore that terrible term, predestination, which hath troubled so many weak heads to conceive, and the wisest to explain, is in respect to God no prescious determination of our estates to come, but a definitive blast of his will already fulfilled, and at the instant that he first decreed it; for, to his eternity, which is indivisible, and altogether, the last trump is already sounded, the reprobates in the flame, and the blessed in Abraham's bosom. St Peter speaks modestly, when he saith, "a thousand years to God are but as one day;" for, to speak like a philosopher, those continued instances of time, which flow into a thousand years, make not to him one moment. What to us is to come, to his eternity is present; his whole duration being but one permanent point, without succession, parts, flux, or division.

§12. — There is no attribute that adds more difficulty to the mystery of the Trinity, where, though in a relative way of Father and Son, we must deny a priority. I wonder how Aristotle could conceive the world eternal, or how he could make good two eternities. His similitude, of a triangle comprehended in a square, doth somewhat illustrate the trinity of our souls, and that the triple unity of God; for there is in us not three, but a trinity of, souls; because there is in us, if not three distinct souls, yet differing faculties, that can and do subsist apart in different subjects, and yet in us are thus united as to make but one soul and substance. If one soul were so perfect as to inform three distinct bodies, that were a pretty trinity. Conceive the distinct number of three, not divided nor separated by the intellect, but actually comprehended in its unity, and that a perfect trinity. I have often admired the mystical way of Pythagoras, and the secret magick of numbers. "Beware of philosophy," is a precept not to be received in too large a sense: for, in this mass of nature, there is a set of things that carry in their front, though not in capital letters, yet in stenography and short characters, something of divinity; which, to wiser reasons, serve as luminaries in the abyss of knowledge, and, to judicious beliefs, as scales and roundles to mount the pinnacles and highest pieces of divinity. The severe schools shall never laugh me out of the philosophy of Hermes, that this visible world is but a picture of the invisible, wherein, as in a portrait, things are not truly, but in equivocal shapes, and as they counterfeit some real substance in that invisible fabrick.

§13. — That other attribute, wherewith I recreate my devotion, is his wisdom, in which I am happy; and for the contemplation of this only do not repent me that I was bred in the way of study. The advantage I have therein, is an ample recompense for all my endeavours, in what part of knowledge soever. Wisdom is his most beauteous attribute: no man can attain unto it: yet Solomon pleased God when he desired it. He is wise, because he knows all things; and he knoweth all things, because he made them all: but his greatest knowledge is in comprehending that he made not, that is, himself. And this is also the greatest knowledge in man. For this do I honour my own profession, and embrace the counsel even of the devil himself: had he read such a lecture in * [Greek omitted] "Nosce teipsum." Paradise as he did at Delphos,*[13] we had better known ourselves; nor had we stood in fear to know him. I know God is wise in all; wonderful in what we conceive, but far more in what we comprehend not: for we behold him but asquint, upon reflex or shadow; our understanding is dimmer than Moses's eye; we are ignorant of the back parts or lower side of his divinity; therefore, to pry into the maze of his counsels, is not only folly in man, but presumption even in angels. Like us, they are his servants, not his senators; he holds no counsel, but that mystical one of the Trinity, wherein, though there be three persons, there is but one mind that decrees without contradiction. Nor needs he any; his actions are not begot with deliberation; his wisdom naturally knows what's best: his intellect stands ready fraught with the superlative and purest ideas of goodness, consultations, and election, which are two motions in us, make but one in him: his actions springing from his power at the first touch of his will. These are contemplations metaphysical: my humble speculations have another method, and are content to trace and discover those expressions he hath left in his creatures, and the obvious effects of nature. There is no danger to profound[14] these mysteries, no *sanctum sanctorum* in philosophy. The world was made to be inhabited by beasts, but studied and contemplated by man: 'tis the debt of our reason we owe unto God, and the homage we pay for not being beasts. Without this, the world is still as though it had not been, or as it was before the sixth day, when as yet there was not a creature that could conceive or say there was a world. The wisdom of God receives small honour from those vulgar heads that rudely stare about, and with a gross rusticity admire his works. Those highly magnify him, whose judicious enquiry into his acts, and deliberate research into his creatures, return the duty of a devout and learned admiration. Therefore,

Search while thou wilt; and let thy reason go,

To ransom truth, e'en to th' abyss below;

Rally the scatter'd causes; and that line

Which nature twists be able to untwine.

It is thy Maker's will; for unto none

But unto reason can he e'er be known.

The devils do know thee; but those damn'd meteors

Build not thy glory, but confound thy creatures.

Teach my endeavours so thy works to read,

That learning them in thee I may proceed.

Give thou my reason that instructive flight,

Whose weary wings may on thy hands still light.

Teach me to soar aloft, yet ever so,

When near the sun, to stoop again below.

Thus shall my humble feathers safely hover,

And, though near earth, more than the heavens discover.

And then at last, when homeward I shall drive,

Rich with the spoils of nature, to my hive,

There will I sit, like that industrious fly,

Buzzing thy praises; which shall never die

Till death abrupts them, and succeeding glory

Bid me go on in a more lasting story.

And this is almost all wherein an humble creature may endeavour to requite, and some way to retribute unto his Creator: for, if not he that saith, "Lord, Lord, but he that doth the will of the Father, shall be saved," certainly our wills must be our performances, and our intents make out our actions; otherwise our pious labours shall find anxiety in our graves, and our best endeavours not hope, but fear, a resurrection.

§14. — There is but one first cause, and four second causes, of all things. Some are without efficient,[15] as God; others without matter, as angels; some without form, as the first matter: but every essence, created or uncreated, hath its final cause, and some positive end both of its essence and operation. This is the cause I grope after in the works of nature; on this hangs the providence of God. To raise so beauteous a structure as the world and the creatures thereof was but his art; but their sundry and divided operations, with their predestinated ends, are from the treasure of his wisdom. In the causes, nature, and affections, of the eclipses of the sun and moon, there is most excellent speculation; but, to profound further, and to contemplate a reason why his providence hath so disposed and ordered their motions in that vast circle, as to conjoin and obscure each other, is a sweeter piece of reason, and a diviner point of philosophy. Therefore, sometimes, and in some things, there appears to me as much divinity in Galen his books, *De Usu Partium*,[16] as in Suarez's Metaphysicks. Had Aristotle been as curious in the enquiry of this cause as he was of the other, he had not left behind him an imperfect piece of philosophy, but an absolute tract of divinity.

§15. — *Natura nihil agit frustra*, is the only indisputable axiom in philosophy. There are no grotesques in nature; not any thing framed to fill up empty cantons, and unnecessary spaces. In the most imperfect creatures, and such as were not preserved in the ark, but, having their seeds and principles in the womb of nature, are everywhere, where the power of the sun is — in these is the wisdom of his hand discovered. Out of this rank Solomon chose the object of his admiration; indeed, what reason may not go to school to the wisdom of bees, ants, and spiders? What wise hand teacheth them to do what reason cannot teach us? Ruder heads stand amazed at those prodigious pieces of nature, whales, elephants, dromedaries, and camels; these, I confess, are the colossus and majestick pieces of her hand; but in these narrow engines there is more curious mathematicks; and the civility of these little citizens more neatly sets forth the wisdom of their Maker. Who admires not Regio Montanus his fly beyond his eagle;[17] or wonders not more at the operation of two souls in those little bodies than but one in the trunk of a cedar? I could never content my contemplation with those general pieces of wonder, the flux and reflux of the sea, the increase of Nile, the conversion of the needle to the north; and have studied to match and parallel those in the more obvious and neglected pieces of nature which, without farther travel, I can do in the cosmography of myself. We carry with us the wonders we seek without us: there is all Africa and her prodigies in us. We are that bold and adventurous piece of nature, which he that studies wisely learns, in a compendium, what others labour at in a divided piece and endless volume.

§16. — Thus there are two books from whence I collect my divinity. Besides that written one of God, another of his servant, nature, that universal and publick manuscript, that lies expansed unto the eyes of all. Those that never saw him in the one have discovered him in the other; this was the scripture and theology of the heathens; the natural motion of the sun made them more admire him than its supernatural station did the children of Israel. The ordinary effects of nature wrought more admiration in them than, in the other, all his miracles. Surely the heathens knew better how to join and read these mystical letters than we Christians, who cast a more careless eye on these common hieroglyphics, and disdain to suck divinity from the flowers of nature. Nor do I so forget God as to adore the name of nature; which I define not, with the schools, to be the principle of motion and rest, but that straight and regular line, that settled and constant course the wisdom of God hath ordained the actions of his creatures, according to their several kinds. To make a revolution every day is the nature of the sun, because of that necessary course which God hath ordained it, from which it cannot swerve but by a faculty from that voice which first did give it motion. Now this course of nature God seldom alters or perverts; but, like an excellent artist, hath so contrived his work, that, with the self-same instrument, without a new creation, he may effect his obscurest designs. Thus he sweeteneth the water with a word, preserveth the creatures in the ark, which the blest of his mouth might have as easily created; — for God is like a skilful geometrician, who, when more easily, and with one stroke of his compass, he might describe or divide a right line, had yet rather do this in a circle or longer way, according to the constituted and forelaid principles of his art: yet this rule of his he doth sometimes pervert, to acquaint the world with his prerogative, lest the arrogancy of our reason should question his power, and conclude he could not. And thus I call the effects of nature the works of God, whose hand and instrument she only is; and therefore, to ascribe his actions unto her is to devolve the honour of the principal agent upon the instrument; which if with reason we may do, then let our hammers rise up and boast they have built our houses, and our pens receive the honour of our writing. I hold there is a general beauty in the works of God, and therefore no deformity in any kind of species of creature whatsoever. I cannot tell by what logick we call a toad, a bear, or an elephant ugly; they being created in those outward shapes and figures which best express the actions of their inward forms; and having passed that general visitation of God, who saw that all that he had made was good, that is, conformable to his will, which abhors deformity, and is the rule of order and beauty. There is no deformity but in monstrosity; wherein, notwithstanding, there is a kind of beauty; nature so ingeniously contriving the irregular part, as they become sometimes more remarkable than the principal fabrick. To speak yet more narrowly, there was never any thing ugly or misshapen, but the chaos; wherein, notwithstanding, to speak strictly, there was no deformity, because no form; nor was it yet impregnant by the voice of God. Now nature is not at variance with art, nor art with nature; they being both the servants of his providence. Art is the perfection of nature. Were the world now as it was the sixth day, there were yet a chaos. Nature hath made one world, and art another. In brief, all things are artificial; for nature is the art of God.

§17. — This is the ordinary and open way of his providence, which art and industry have in good part discovered; whose effects we may foretell without an oracle. To foreshow these is not prophecy, but prognostication. There is another way, full of meanders and labyrinths, whereof the devil and spirits have no exact ephemerides: and that is a more particular and obscure method of his providence; directing the operations of individual and single essences: this we call fortune; that serpentine and crooked line, whereby he draws those actions his wisdom intends in a more unknown and secret way; this cryptic[18] and involved

17

method of his providence have I ever admired; nor can I relate the history of my life, the occurrences of my days, the escapes, or dangers, and hits of chance, with a *bezo las manos* to Fortune, or a bare gramercy to my good stars. Abraham might have thought the ram in the thicket came thither by accident: human reason would have said that mere chance conveyed Moses in the ark to the sight of Pharaoh's daughter. What a labyrinth is there in the story of Joseph! able to convert a stoick. Surely there are in every man's life certain rubs, doublings, and wrenches, which pass a while under the effects of chance; but at the last, well examined, prove the mere hand of God. 'Twas not dumb chance that, to discover the fougade,[19] or powder plot, contrived a miscarriage in the letter. I like the victory of '88[20] the better for that one occurrence which our enemies imputed to our dishonour, and the partiality of fortune; to wit, the tempests and contrariety of winds. King Philip did not detract from the nation, when he said, he sent his armada to fight with men, and not to combat with the winds. Where there is a manifest disproportion between the powers and forces of two several agents, upon a maxim of reason we may promise the victory to the superior: but when unexpected accidents slip in, and unthought-of occurrences intervene, these must proceed from a power that owes no obedience to those axioms; where, as in the writing upon the wall, we may behold the hand, but see not the spring that moves it. The success of that petty province of Holland (of which the Grand Seignior proudly said, if they should trouble him, as they did the Spaniard, he would send his men with shovels and pickaxes, and throw it into the sea) I cannot altogether ascribe to the ingenuity and industry of the people, but the mercy of God, that hath disposed them to such a thriving genius; and to the will of his providence, that disposeth her favour to each country in their preordinate season. All cannot be happy at once; for, because the glory of one state depends upon the ruin of another, there is a revolution and vicissitude of their greatness, and must obey the swing of that wheel, not moved by intelligencies, but by the hand of God, whereby all estates arise to their zenith and vertical points, according to their predestinated periods. For the lives, not only of men, but of commonwealths and the whole world, run not upon a helix that still enlargeth; but on a circle, where, arriving to their meridian, they decline in obscurity, and fall under the horizon again.

§18. — These must not therefore be named the effects of fortune but in a relative way, and as we term the works of nature. It was the ignorance of man's reason that begat this very name, and by a careless term miscalled the providence of God: for there is no liberty for causes to operate in a loose and straggling way; nor any effect whatsoever but hath its warrant from some universal or superior cause. 'Tis not a ridiculous devotion to say a prayer before a game at tables; for, even in sortileges[21] and matters of greatest uncertainty, there is a settled and preordered course of effects. It is we that are blind, not fortune. Because our eye is too dim to discover the mystery of her effects, we foolishly paint her blind, and hoodwink the providence of the Almighty. I cannot justify that con temptible proverb, that "fools only are fortunate;" or that insolent paradox, that "a wise man is out of the reach of fortune;" much less those opprobrious epithets of poets — "whore," "bawd," and "strumpet." 'Tis, I confess, the common fate of men of singular gifts of mind, to be destitute of those of fortune; which doth not any way deject the spirit of wiser judgments who thoroughly understand the justice of this proceeding; and, being enriched with higher donatives, cast a more careless eye on these vulgar parts of felicity. It is a most unjust ambition, to desire to engross the mercies of the Almighty, not to be content with the goods of mind, without a possession of those of body or fortune: and it is an error, worse than heresy, to adore these complimental and circumstantial pieces of felicity, and undervalue those perfections and essential points of happiness, wherein we resemble our Maker. To wiser desires it is satisfaction enough to deserve, though not to enjoy, the favours of fortune. Let providence provide for fools: 'tis not partiality, but equity, in God, who deals with us but as our natural parents. Those that are able of body and mind he leaves to their deserts; to those of weaker merits he imparts a larger portion; and pieces out the defect of one by the excess of the other. Thus have we no just quarrel with nature for leaving us naked; or to envy the horns, hoofs, skins, and furs of other creatures; being provided with reason, that can supply them all. We need not labour, with so many arguments, to confute judicial astrology; for, if there be a truth therein, it doth not injure divinity. If to be born under Mercury disposeth us to be witty; under Jupiter to be wealthy; I do not owe a knee unto these, but unto that merciful hand that hath ordered my indifferent and uncertain nativity unto such benevolous aspects. Those that hold that all things are governed by fortune, had not erred, had they not persisted there. The Romans, that erected a temple to Fortune, acknowledged therein, though in a blinder way, somewhat of divinity; for, in a wise supputation,[22] all things begin and end in the Almighty. There is a nearer way to heaven than Homer's chain;[23] an easy logick may conjoin a heaven and earth in one argument, and, with less than a sorites,[24] resolve all things to God. For though we christen effects by their most sensible and nearest causes, yet is God the true and infallible cause of all; whose concourse, though it be general, yet doth it subdivide itself into the particular actions of every thing, and is that spirit, by which each singular essence not only subsists, but performs its operation.

§19. — The bad construction and perverse comment on these pair of second causes, or visible hands of God, have perverted the devotion of many unto atheism; who, forgetting the honest advisoes of faith, have listened unto the conspiracy of passion and reason. I have therefore always endeavoured to compose those feuds and angry dissensions between affection, faith, and reason: for there is in our soul a kind of triumvirate, or triple government of three competitors, which distracts the peace of this our commonwealth not less than did that other[25] the state of Rome.

As reason is a rebel unto faith, so passion unto reason. As the propositions of faith seem absurd unto reason, so the theorems of reason unto passion and both unto reason; yet a moderate and peaceable discretion may so state and order the matter, that they may be all kings, and yet make but one monarchy: every one exercising his sovereignty and prerogative in a due time and place, according to the restraint and limit of circumstance. There are, as in philosophy, so in divinity, sturdy doubts, and boisterous objections, wherewith the unhappiness of our knowledge too nearly acquainteth us. More of these no man hath known than myself; which I confess I conquered, not in a martial posture, but on my knees. For our endeavours are not only to combat with doubts, but always to dispute with the devil. The villany of that spirit takes a hint of infidelity from our studios; and, by demonstrating a naturality in one way, makes us mistrust a miracle in another. Thus, having perused the Archidoxes, and read the secret sympathies of things, he would dissuade my belief from the miracle of the brazen serpent; make me conceit that image worked by sympathy, and was but an Egyptian trick, to cure their diseases without a miracle. Again, having seen some experiments of bitumen, and having read far more of naphtha, he whispered to my curiosity the fire of the altar might be natural, and bade me mistrust a miracle in Elias, when he intrenched the altar round with water: for that inflamable substance yields not easily unto water, but flames in the arms of its antagonist. And thus would he inveigle my belief to think the combustion of Sodom might be natural, and that there was an asphaltick and bituminous nature in that lake before the fire of Gomorrah. I know that manna is now plentifully gathered in Calabria; and Josephus tells me, in his days it was as plentiful in Arabia. The devil therefore made the query, "Where was then the miracle in the days of Moses?" The Israelites saw but that, in his time, which the natives of those countries behold in ours. Thus the devil played at chess with me, and, yielding a pawn, thought to gain a queen of me; taking advantage of my honest endeavours; and, whilst I laboured to raise the structure of my reason, he strove to undermine the edifice of my faith.

20

§20. — Neither had these or any other ever such advantage of me, as to incline me to any point of infidelity or desperate positions of atheism; for I have been these many years of opinion there was never any. Those that held religion was the difference of man from beasts, have spoken probably, and proceed upon a principle as inductive as the other. That doctrine of Epicurus, that denied the providence of God, was no atheism, but a magnificent and high-strained conceit of his majesty, which he deemed too sublime to mind the trivial actions of those inferior creatures. That fatal necessity of the stoicks is nothing but the immutable law of his will. Those that heretofore denied the divinity of the Holy Ghost have been condemned but as hereticks; and those that now deny our Saviour, though more than hereticks, are not so much as atheists: for, though they deny two persons in the Trinity, they hold, as we do, there is but one God.

That villain and secretary of hell,[26] that composed that miscreant piece of the three impostors, though divided from all religions, and neither Jew, Turk, nor Christian, was not a positive atheist. I confess every country hath its Machiavel, every age its Lucian, whereof common heads must not hear, nor more advanced judgments too rashly venture on. It is the rhetorick of Satan; and may pervert a loose or prejudicate belief.

§21. — I confess I have perused them all, and can discover nothing that may startle a discreet belief; yet are their heads carried off with the wind and breath of such motives. I remember a doctor in physick, of Italy, who could not perfectly believe the immortality of the soul, because Galen seemed to make a doubt thereof. With another I was familiarly acquainted, in France, a divine, and a man of singular parts, that on the same point was * "Post mortem nihil est, ipsaque mors nihil, mors individua est noxia corpori, nec patiens animae. . . . Toti morimur nullaque pars manet nostri." so plunged and gravelled with three lines of Seneca,* that all our antidotes, drawn from both Scripture and philosophy, could not expel the poison of his error. There are a set of heads that can credit the relations of mariners, yet question the testimonies of Saint Paul: and peremptorily maintain the traditions of Ælian or Pliny; yet, in histories of Scripture, raise queries and objections: believing no more than they can parallel in human authors. I confess there are, in Scripture, stories that do exceed the fables of poets, and, to a captious reader, sound like Garagantua or Bevis. Search all the legends of times past, and the fabulous conceits of these present, and 'twill be hard to find one that deserves to carry the buckler unto Samson; yet is all this of an easy possibility, if we conceive a divine concourse, or an influence from the little finger of the Almighty. It is impossible that, either in the discourse of man or in the infallible voice of God, to the weakness of our apprehensions there should not appear irregularities, contradictions, and antinomies:[27] myself could show a catalogue of doubts, never yet imagined nor questioned, as I know, which are not resolved at the first hearing; not fantastick queries or objections of air; for I cannot hear of atoms in divinity. I can read the history of the pigeon that was sent out of the ark, and returned no more, yet not question how she found out her mate that was left behind: that Lazarus was raised from the dead, yet not demand where, in the interim, his soul awaited; or raise a lawcase, whether his heir might lawfully detain his inheritance bequeathed upon him by his death, and he, though restored to life, have no plea or title unto his former possessions. Whether Eve was framed out of the left side of Adam, I dispute not; because I stand not yet assured which is the right side of a man; or whether there be any such distinction in nature. That she was edified out of the rib of Adam, I believe; yet raise no question who shall arise with that rib at the resurrection. Whether Adam was an hermaphrodite, as the rabbins contend upon the letter of the text; because it is contrary to reason, there should be an hermaphrodite before there was a woman, or a composition of two natures, before there was a second composed. Likewise, whether the world was created in autumn, summer, or the spring; because it was created in them all: for, whatsoever sign the sun possesseth, those four seasons are actually existent. It is the nature of this luminary to distinguish the several seasons of the year; all which it makes at one time in the whole earth, and successively in any part thereof. There are a bundle of curiosities, not only in philosophy, but in divinity, proposed and discussed by men of most supposed abilities, which indeed are not worthy our vacant hours, * In Rabelais. much less our serious studies. Pieces only fit to be placed in Pantagruel's library,[28] or bound up with Tartaratus, *De Modo Cacandi.*[29]

§22. — These are niceties that become not those that peruse so serious a mystery. There are others more generally questioned, and called to the bar, yet, methinks, of an easy and possible truth.

'Tis ridiculous to put off or down the general flood of Noah, in that particular inundation of Deucalion.[30] That there was a deluge once seems not to me so great a miracle as that there is not one always. How all the kinds of creatures, not only in their own bulks, but with a competency of food and sustenance, might be preserved in one ark, and within the extent of three hundred cubits, to a reason that rightly examines it, will appear very feasible. There is another secret, not contained in the Scripture, which is more hard to comprehend, and put the honest Father[31] to the refuge of a miracle; and that is, not only how the distinct pieces of the world, and divided islands, should be first planted by men, but inhabited by tigers, panthers, and bears. How America abounded with beasts of prey, and noxious animals, yet contained not in it that necessary creature, a horse, is very strange. By what passage those, not only birds, but dangerous and unwelcome beasts, come over. How there be creatures there (which are not found in this triple continent). All which must needs be strange unto us, that hold but one ark; and that the creatures began their progress from the mountains of Ararat. They who, to salve this, would make the deluge particular, proceed upon a principle that I can no way grant; not only upon the negative of Holy Scriptures, but of mine own reason, whereby I can make it probable that the world was as well peopled in the time of Noah as in ours; and fifteen hundred years, to people the world, as full a time for them as four thousand years since have been to us. There are other assertions and common tenets drawn from Scripture, and generally believed as Scripture, whereunto, notwithstanding, I would never betray the liberty of my reason. 'Tis a paradox to me, that Methusalem was the longest lived of all the children of Adam; and no man will be able to prove it; when, from the process of the text, I can manifest it may be otherwise. That Judas perished by hanging himself, there is no certainty in Scripture: though, in one place, it seems to affirm it, and, by a doubtful word, hath given occasion to translate[32] it; yet, in another place, in a more punctual description, it makes it improbable, and seems to overthrow it. That our fathers, after the flood, erected the tower of Babel, to preserve themselves against a second deluge, is generally opinioned and believed; yet is there another intention of theirs expressed in Scripture. Besides, it is improbable, from the circumstance of the place; that is, a plain in the land of Shinar. These are no points of faith; and therefore may admit a free dispute. There are yet others, and those familiarly concluded from the text, wherein (under favour) I see no consequence. The church of Rome confidently proves the opinion of tutelary angels, from that answer, when Peter knocked at the door, "'Tis not he, but his angel;" that is, might some say, his messenger, or somebody from him; for so the original signifies; and is as likely to be the doubtful family's meaning. This exposition I once suggested to a young divine, that answered upon this point; to which I remember the Franciscan opponent replied no more, but, that it was a new, and no authentick interpretation.

§23. — These are but the conclusions and fallible discourses of man upon the word of God; for such I do believe the Holy Scriptures; yet, were it of man, I could not choose but say, it was the singularest and superlative

23

piece that hath been extant since the creation. Were I a pagan, I should not refrain the lecture of it; and cannot but commend the judgment of Ptolemy, that thought not his library complete without it. The Alcoran of the Turks (I speak without prejudice) is an ill-composed piece, containing in it vain and ridiculous errors in philosophy, impossibilities, fictions, and vanities beyond laughter, maintained by evident and open sophisms, the policy of ignorance, deposition of universities, and banishment of learning. That hath gotten foot by arms and violence: this, without a blow, hath disseminated itself through the whole earth. It is not unremarkable, what Philo first observed, that the law of Moses continued two thousand years without the least alteration; whereas, we see, the laws of other commonwealths do alter with occasions: and even those, that pretended their original from some divinity, to have vanished without trace or memory. I believe, besides Zoroaster, there were divers others that writ before Moses; who, notwithstanding, have suffered the common fate of time. Men's works have an age, like themselves; and though they outlive their authors, yet have they a stint and period to their duration. This only is a work too hard for the teeth of time, and cannot perish but in the general flames, when all things shall confess their ashes.

§24. — I have heard some with deep sighs lament the lost lines of Cicero; others with as many groans deplore the combustion of the library of Alexandria;[33] for my own part, I think there be too many in the world; and could with patience behold the urn and ashes of the Vatican, could I, with a few others, recover the perished leaves of Solomon. I would not omit a copy of Enoch's pillars,[34] had they many nearer authors than Josephus, or did not relish somewhat of the fable. Some men have written more than others have spoken. Pineda * Pineda, in his "Monarchia Ecclesiastica," quotes one thousand and forty authors. [35] quotes more authors, in one work,* than are necessary in a whole world. Of those three great inventions in Germany,[36] there are two which are not without their incommodities, and 'tis disputable whether they exceed not their use and commodities. 'Tis not a melancholy *utinam* of my own, but the desires of better heads, that there were a general synod — not to unite the incompatible difference of religion, but — for the benefit of learning, to reduce it, as it lay at first, in a few and solid authors; and to condemn to the fire those swarms and millions of rhapsodies, begotten only to distract and abuse the weaker judgments of scholars, and to maintain the trade and mystery of typographers.

§25. — I cannot but wonder with what exception the Samaritans could confine their belief to the Pentateuch, or five books of Moses. I am ashamed at the rabbinical interpretation of the Jews upon the Old Testament,[37] as much as their defection from the New: and truly it is beyond wonder, how that contemptible and degenerate issue of Jacob, once so devoted to ethnick superstition, and so easily seduced to the idolatry of their neighbours, should now, in such an obstinate and peremptory belief, adhere unto their own doctrine, expect impossibilities, and in the face and eye of the church, persist without the least hope of conversion. This is a vice in them, that were a virtue in us; for obstinacy in a bad cause is but constancy in a good: and herein I must accuse those of my own religion; for there is not any of such a fugitive faith, such an unstable belief, as a Christian; none that do so often transform themselves, not unto several shapes of Christianity, and of the same species, but unto more unnatural and contrary forms of Jew and Mohammedan; that, from the name of Saviour, can condescend to the bare term of prophet: and, from an old belief that he is come, fall to a new expectation of his coming. It is the promise of Christ, to make us all one flock: but how and when this union shall be, is as obscure to me as the last day. Of those four members of religion we hold a slender proportion.[38] There are, I confess, some new additions; yet small to those which accrue to our adversaries; and those only drawn from the revolt of pagans; men but of negative impieties; and such as deny Christ, but because they never heard of him. But the religion of the Jew is expressly against the Christian, and the Mohammedan against both; for the Turk, in the bulk he now stands, is beyond all hope of conversion: if he fall asunder, there may be conceived hopes; but not without strong improbabilities. The Jew is obstinate in all fortunes; the persecution of fifteen hundred years hath but confirmed them in their error. They have already endured whatsoever may be inflicted: and have suffered, in a bad cause, even to the condemnation of their enemies. Persecution is a bad and indirect way to plant religion. It hath been the unhappy method of angry devotions, not only to confirm honest religion, but wicked heresies and extravagant opinions. It was the first stone and basis of our faith. None can more justly boast of persecutions, and glory in the number and valour of martyrs. For, to speak properly, those are true and almost only examples of fortitude. Those that are fetched from the field, or drawn from the actions of the camp, are not ofttimes so truly precedents of valour as audacity, and, at the best, attain but to some bastard piece of fortitude. If we shall strictly examine the circumstances and requisites which Aristotle requires[39] to true and perfect valour, we shall find the name only in his master, Alexander, and as little in that Roman worthy, Julius Caesar; and if any, in that easy and active way, have done so nobly as to deserve that name, yet, in the passive and more terrible piece, these have surpassed, and in a more heroical way

25

may claim, the honour of that title. 'Tis not in the power of every honest faith to proceed thus far, or pass to heaven through the flames. Every one hath it not in that full measure, nor in so audacious and resolute a temper, as to endure those terrible tests and trials; who, notwithstanding, in a peaceable way, do truly adore their Saviour, and have, no doubt, a faith acceptable in the eyes of God.

§26. — Now, as all that die in the war are not termed soldiers, so neither can I properly term all those that suffer in matters of religion, martyrs. The council of Constance condemns John Huss for a heretick;[40] the stories of his own party style him a martyr. He must needs offend the divinity of both, that says he was neither the one nor the other. There are many (questionless) canonized on earth, that shall never be saints in heaven; and have their names in histories and martyrologies, who, in the eyes of God, are not so perfect martyrs as was that wise heathen Socrates, that suffered on a fundamental point of religion — the unity of God. I have often pitied the miserable bishop[41] that suffered in the cause of antipodes; yet cannot choose but accuse him of as much madness, for exposing his living on such a trifle, as those of ignorance and folly, that condemned him. I think my conscience will not give me the lie, if I say there are not many extant, that, in a noble way, fear the face of death less than myself; yet, from the moral duty I owe to the commandment of God, and the natural respect that I tender unto the conservation of my essence and being, I would not perish upon a ceremony, politick points, or indifferency: nor is my belief of that untractable temper as, not to bow at their obstacles, or connive at matters wherein there are not manifest impieties. The leaven, therefore, and ferment of all, not only civil, but religious, actions, is wisdom; without which, to commit ourselves to the flames is homicide, and (I fear) but to pass through one fire into another.

§27. — That miracles are ceased, I can neither prove nor absolutely deny, much less define the time and period of their cessation. That they survived Christ is manifest upon record of Scripture: that they outlived the apostles also, and were revived at the conversion of nations, many years after, we cannot deny, if we shall not question those writers whose testimonies we do not controvert in points that make for our own opinions: therefore, that may have some truth in it, that is reported by the Jesuits of their miracles in the Indies. I could wish it were true, or had any other testimony than their own pens. They may easily believe those miracles abroad, who daily conceive a greater at home — the transmutation of those visible elements into the body and blood of our Saviour; — for the conversion of water into wine, which he wrought in

Cana, or, what the devil would have had him done in the wilderness, of stones into bread, compared to this, will scarce deserve the name of a miracle: though, indeed, to speak properly, there is not one miracle greater than another; they being the extraordinary effects of the hand of God, to which all things are of an equal facility; and to create the world as easy as one single creature. For this is also a miracle; not only to produce effects against or above nature, but before nature; and to create nature, as great a miracle as to contradict or transcend her. We do too narrowly define the power of God, restraining it to our capacities. I hold that God can do all things: how he should work contradictions, I do not understand, yet dare not, therefore, deny. I cannot see why the angel of God should question Esdras to recall the time past, if it were beyond his own power; or that God should pose mortality in that which he was not able to perform himself. I will not say that God cannot, but he will not, perform many things, which we plainly affirm he cannot. This, I am sure, is the mannerliest proposition; wherein, notwithstanding, I hold no paradox: for, strictly, his power is the same with his will; and they both, with all the rest, do make but one God.

§28. — Therefore, that miracles have been, I do believe; that they may yet be wrought by the living, I do not deny: but have no confidence in those which are fathered on the dead. And this hath ever made me suspect the efficacy of relicks, to examine the bones, question the habits and appertenances of saints, and even of Christ himself. I cannot conceive why the cross that Helena[42] found, and whereon Christ himself died, should have power to restore others unto life. I excuse not Constantine from a fall off his horse, or a mischief from his enemies, upon the wearing those nails on his bridle which our Saviour bore upon the cross in his hands. I compute among *piae fraudes*, nor many degrees before consecrated swords and roses, that which Baldwin, king of Jerusalem, returned the Genoese for their costs and pains in his wars; to wit, the ashes of John the Baptist. Those that hold, the sanctity of their souls doth leave behind a tincture and sacred faculty on their bodies, speak naturally of miracles, and do not salve the doubt. Now, one reason I tender so little devotion unto relicks is, I think the slender and doubtful respect which I have always held unto antiquities. For that, indeed, which I admire, is far before antiquity; that is, Eternity; and that is, God himself; who, though he be styled the Ancient of Days, cannot receive the adjunct of antiquity, who was before the world, and shall be after it, yet is not older than it: for, in his years there is no climacter:[43] his duration is eternity; and far more venerable than antiquity.

§29. — But, above all things, I wonder how the curiosity of wiser heads could pass that great and indisputable miracle, the cessation of oracles; and in what swoon their reasons lay, to content themselves, and sit down with such a far-fetched and ridiculous reason as Plutarch allegeth for it.[44] The Jews, that can believe the supernatural solstice of the sun in the days of Joshua, have yet the impudence to deny the eclipse, which every pagan confessed, at his death; but for this, it is evident beyond all contradiction: * In his oracle to Augustus. the devil himself confessed it.* Certainly it is not a warrantable curiosity, to examine the verity of Scripture by the concordance of human history; or seek to confirm the chronicle of Hester or Daniel by the authority of Megasthenes[45] or Herodotus. I confess, I have had an un happy curiosity this way, till I laughed myself out of it with a piece of Justin, where he delivers that the children of Israel, for being scabbed, were banished out of Egypt. And truly, since I have understood the occurrences of the world, and know in what counterfeiting shapes and deceitful visards times present represent on the stage things past, I do believe them little more than things to come. Some have been of my own opinion, and endeavoured to write the history of their own lives; wherein Moses hath outgone them all, and left not only the story of his life, but, as some will have it, of his death also.

§30. — It is a riddle to me, how the story of oracles hath not wormed out of the world that doubtful conceit of spirits and witches; how so many learned heads should so far forget their metaphysicks, and destroy the ladder and scale of creatures, as to question the existence of spirits; for my part, I have ever believed, and do now know, that there are witches. They that doubt of these do not only deny them, but spirits: and are obliquely, and upon consequence, a sort, not of infidels, but atheists. Those that, to confute their incredulity, desire to see apparitions, shall, questionless, never behold any, nor have the power to be so much as witches. The devil hath made them already in a heresy as capital as witchcraft; and to appear to them were but to convert them. Of all the delusions wherewith he deceives mortality, there is not any that puzzleth me more than the legerdemain of changelings.[46] I do not credit those transformations of reasonable creatures into beasts, or that the devil hath a power to transpeciate a man into a horse, who tempted Christ (as a trial of his divinity) to convert but stones into bread. I could believe that spirits use with man the act of carnality; and that in both sexes. I conceive they may assume, steal, or contrive a body, wherein there may be action enough to content decrepit lust, or passion to satisfy more active veneries; yet, in both, without a possibility of generation: and therefore that opinion, that Antichrist should be born of the tribe of Dan, by conjunction with the

28

devil, is ridiculous, and a conceit fitter for a rabbin than a Christian. I hold that the devil doth really possess some men; the spirit of melancholy others; the spirit of delusion others: that, as the devil is concealed and denied by some, so God and good angels are pretended by others, whereof the late defection of the maid of Germany hath left a pregnant example.[47]

§31. — Again, I believe that all that use sorceries, incantations, and spells, are not witches, or, as we term them, magicians. I conceive there is a traditional magick, not learned immediately from the devil, but at second hand from his scholars, who, having once the secret betrayed, are able and do empirically practise without his advice; they both proceeding upon the principles of nature; where actives, aptly conjoined to disposed passives, will, under any master, produce their effects. Thus, I think, at first, a great part of philosophy was witchcraft; which, being afterward derived to one another, proved but philosophy, and was indeed no more than the honest effects of nature:— what invented by us, is philosophy; learned from him, is magick. We do surely owe the discovery of many secrets to the discovery of good and bad angels. I could never pass that sentence of Paracelsus * Thereby is meant our good angel, appointed us from our nativity. without an asterisk, or annotation: "ascendens* constellatum multa revelat quaerentibus magnalia naturae, i.e. *opera Dei.*" I do think that many mysteries ascribed to our own inventions have been the corteous revelations of spirits; for those noble essences in heaven bear a friendly regard unto their fellow-nature on earth; and therefore believe that those many prodigies and ominous prognosticks, which forerun the ruins of states, princes, and private persons, are the charitable premonitions of good angels, which more careless inquiries term but the effects of chance and nature.

§32. — Now, besides these particular and divided spirits, there may be (for aught I know) a universal and common spirit to the whole world. It was the opinion of Plato, and is yet of the hermetical philosophers. If there be a common nature, that unites and ties the scattered and divided individuals into one species, why may there not be one that unites them all? However, I am sure there is a common spirit, that plays within us, yet makes no part in us; and that is, the spirit of God; the fire and scintillation of that noble and mighty essence, which is the life and radical heat of spirits, and those essences that know not the virtue of the sun; a fire quite contrary to the fire of hell. This is that gentle heat that brooded on the waters, and in six days hatched the world; this is that irradiation that dispels the mists of hell, the clouds of horror, fear, sorrow, despair; and preserves the region of the mind in serenity. Whatsoever feels not the warm gale and gentle ventilation of this spirit (though I feel his pulse), I dare not say he lives; for truly without this, to me, there is no heat under the tropick; nor any light, though I dwelt in the body of the sun.

"As when the labouring sun hath wrought his track

Up to the top of lofty Cancer's back,

The icy ocean cracks, the frozen pole

Thaws with the heat of the celestial coal;

So when thy absent beams begin t'impart

Again a solstice on my frozen heart,

My winter's o'er, my drooping spirits sing,

And every part revives into a spring.

But if thy quickening beams a while decline,

And with their light bless not this orb of mine,

A chilly frost surpriseth every member.

And in the midst of June I feel December.

Oh how this earthly temper doth debase

The noble soul, in this her humble place!

Whose wingy nature ever doth aspire

To reach that place whence first it took its fire.

These flames I feel, which in my heart do dwell,

Are not thy beams, but take their fire from hell.

Oh quench them all! and let thy Light divine

Be as the sun to this poor orb of mine!

And to thy sacred Spirit convert those fires,

Whose earthly fumes choke my devout aspires!"

§33. — Therefore, for spirits, I am so far from denying their existence, that I could easily believe, that not only whole countries, but particular persons, have their tutelary and guardian angels. It is not a new opinion of the Church of Rome, but an old one of Pythagoras and Plato: there is no heresy in it: and if not manifestly defined in Scripture, yet it is an opinion of a good and wholesome use in the course and actions of a man's life; and would serve as an hypothesis to salve many doubts, whereof common philosophy affordeth no solution. Now, if you demand my opinion and metaphysicks of their natures, I confess them very shallow; most of them in a negative way, like that of God; or in a comparative, between ourselves and fellow-creatures: for there is in this universe a stair, or manifest scale, of creatures, rising not disorderly, or in confusion, but with a comely method and proportion. Between creatures of mere existence and things of life there is a large disproportion of nature: between plants and animals, or creatures of sense, a wider difference: between them and man, a far greater: and if the proportion hold on, between man and angels there should be yet a greater. We do not comprehend their natures, who retain the first definition of Porphyry;[48] and distinguish them from ourselves by immortality: for, before his fall, man also was immortal: yet must we needs affirm that he had a different essence from the angels. Having, therefore, no certain knowledge of their nature, 'tis no bad method of the schools, whatsoever perfection we find obscurely in ourselves, in a more complete and absolute way to ascribe unto them. I believe they have an extemporary knowledge, and, upon the first motion of their reason, do what we cannot without study or deliberation: that they know things by their forms, and define, by specifical difference what we describe by accidents and properties: and therefore probabilities to us may be demonstrations unto them: that they have knowledge not only of the specifical, but numerical, forms of individuals, and understand by what reserved difference each single hypostatis (besides the relation to its species) becomes its numerical self: that, as the soul hath a power to move the body it informs, so there's a faculty to move any, though inform none: ours upon restraint of time, place, and distance: but that invisible hand that conveyed Habakkuk to the lion's den, or Philip to Azotus, infringeth this rule, and hath a secret conveyance, wherewith mortality is not acquainted. If they have that intuitive knowledge, whereby, as in reflection, they behold the thoughts of one another, I cannot peremptorily deny but they know a great part of ours. They that, to refute the invocation of saints, have denied that they have any knowledge of our affairs below, have proceeded too far, and must pardon my opinion, till I can thoroughly answer that piece of Scripture, "At the conversion of a sinner, the angels in heaven rejoice." I cannot, with those in that great father,[49] securely interpret the work of the first day, *fiat lux*, to the creation of angels; though I confess there is not any creature that hath so near a glimpse of their nature as light in the sun and elements: we style it a bare accident; but, where it subsists alone, 'tis a spiritual substance, and may be an angel: in brief, conceive light invisible, and that is a spirit.

§34. — These are certainly the magisterial and masterpieces of the Creator; the flower, or, as we may say, the best part of nothing; actually existing, what we are but in hopes, and probability. We are only that amphibious piece, between a corporeal and a spiritual essence; that middle form, that links those two together, and makes good the method of God and nature, that jumps not from extremes, but unites the incompatible distances by some middle and participating natures. That we are the breath and similitude of God, it is indisputable, and upon record of Holy Scripture: but to call ourselves a microcosm, or little world, I thought it only a pleasant trope of rhetorick, till my near judgment and second thoughts told me there was a real truth therein. For, first we are a rude mass, and in the rank of creatures which only are, and have a dull kind of being, not yet privileged with life, or preferred to sense or reason; next we live the life of plants, the life of animals, the life of men, and at last the life of spirits: running on, in one mysterious nature, those five kinds of existencies, which comprehend the creatures, not only of the world, but of the universe. Thus is man that great and true *amphibium*, whose nature is disposed to live, not only like other creatures in divers elements, but in divided and distinguished worlds; for though there be but one to sense, there are two to reason, the one visible, the other invisible; whereof Moses seems to have left description, and of the other so obscurely, that some parts thereof are yet in controversy. And truly, for the first chapters of Genesis, I must confess a great deal of obscurity; though divines have, to the power of human reason, endeavoured to make all go in a literal meaning, yet those allegorical interpretations are also probable, and perhaps the mystical method of Moses, bred up in the hieroglyphical schools of the Egyptians.

§35. — Now for that immaterial world, methinks we need not wander so far as the first moveable; for, even in this material fabrick, the spirits walk as freely exempt from the affection of time, place, and motion, as beyond the extremest circumference. Do but extract from the corpulency of bodies, or resolve things beyond their first matter, and you discover the habitation of angels; which if I call the ubiquitary and omnipresent essence of God, I hope I shall not offend divinity: for, before the creation of the world, God was really all things. For the angels he created no new world, or determinate mansion, and therefore they are everywhere where is his essence, and do live, at a distance even, in himself. That God made all things for man, is in some sense true; yet, not so far as to subordinate the creation of those purer creatures unto ours; though, as ministering spirits, they do, and are willing to fulfil the will of God in these lower and sublunary affairs of man. God made all things for himself; and it is impossible he should make them for any other end than his own glory: it is all he can receive, and all that is without himself. For, honour being an external adjunct, and in the honourer rather than in the person honoured, it was necessary to make a creature, from whom he might receive this homage: and that is, in the other world, angels, in this, man; which when we neglect, we forget God, not only to repent that he hath made the world, but that he hath sworn he would not destroy it. That there is but one world, is a conclusion of faith; Aristotle with all his philosophy hath not been able to prove it: and as weakly that the world was eternal; that dispute much troubled the pen of the philosophers, but Moses decided that question, and all is salved with the new term of a creation — that is, a production of something out of nothing. And what is that? — whatsoever is opposite to something; or, more exactly, that which is truly contrary unto God: for he only is; all others have an existence with dependency, and are something but by a distinction. And herein is divinity conformant unto philosophy, and generation not only founded on contrarieties, but also creation. God, being all things, is contrary unto nothing; out of which were made all things, and so nothing became something, and omneity[50] informed nullity into an essence.

§36. — The whole creation is a mystery, and particularly that of man. At the blast of his mouth were the rest of the creatures made; and at his bare word they started out of nothing: but in the frame of man (as the text describes it) he played the sensible operator, and seemed not so much to create as make him. When he had separated the materials of other creatures, there consequently resulted a form and soul; but, having raised the walls of man, he was driven to a second and harder creation — of a substance like himself, an incorruptible and immortal soul. For these two affections we have the philosophy and opinion of the heathens, the flat affirmative of Plato, and not a negative from Aristotle. There is another scruple cast in by divinity concerning its production, much disputed in the German auditories, and with that indifference and equality of arguments, as leave the controversy undetermined. I am not of Paracelsus's mind, that boldly delivers a receipt to make a man without conjunction; yet cannot but wonder at the multitude of heads that do deny traduction, having no other arguments to confirm their belief than that rhetorical sentence and *antimetathesis*[51] of Augustine, "creando infunditur, infundendo creatur." Either opinion will consist well enough with religion: yet I should rather incline to this, did not one objection haunt me, not wrung from speculations and subtleties, but from common sense and observation; not pick'd from the leaves of any author, but bred amongst the weeds and tares of my own brain. And this is a conclusion from the equivocal and monstrous productions in the copulation of a man with a beast: for if the soul of man be not transmitted and transfused in the seed of the parents, why are not those productions merely beasts, but have also an impression and tincture of reason in as high a measure, as it can evidence itself in those improper organs? Nor, truly, can I peremptorily deny that the soul, in this her sublunary estate, is wholly, and in all acceptions, inorganical: but that, for the performance of her ordinary actions, is required not only a symmetry and proper disposition of organs, but a crasis and temper correspondent to its operations; yet is not this mass of flesh and visible structure the instrument and proper corpse of the soul, but rather of sense, and that the hand of reason. In our study of anatomy there is a mass of mysterious philosophy, and such as reduced the very heathens to divinity; yet, amongst all those rare discoveries and curious pieces I find in the fabrick of man, I do not so much content myself, as in that I find not — that is, no organ or instrument for the rational soul; for in the brain, which we term the seat of reason, there is not anything of moment more than I can discover in the crany of a beast; and this is a sensible and no inconsiderable argument of the inorganity of the soul, at least in that sense we usually so conceive it. Thus we are men, and we know not how; there is something in us that can be without us, and will be after us, though it is strange that it hath no history what it was before us, nor cannot tell how it entered in us.

$37. — Now, for these walls of flesh, wherein the soul doth seem to be immured before the resurrection, it is nothing but an elemental composition, and a fabrick that must fall to ashes. "All flesh is grass," is not only metaphorically, but literally, true; for all those creatures we behold are but the herbs of the field, digested into flesh in them, or more remotely carnified in ourselves. Nay, further, we are what we all abhor, *anthropophagi*, and cannibals, devourers not only of men, but of ourselves;

34

and that not in an allegory but a positive truth: for all this mass of flesh which we behold, came in at our mouths: this frame we look upon, hath been upon our trenchers; in brief, we have devoured ourselves. I cannot believe the wisdom of Pythagoras did ever positively, and in a literal sense, affirm his metempsychosis, or impossible transmigration of the souls of men into beasts. Of all metamorphoses or transmigrations, I believe only one, that is of Lot's wife; for that of Nabuchodonosor proceeded not so far. In all others I conceive there is no further verity than is contained in their implicit sense and morality. I believe that the whole frame of a beast doth perish, and is left in the same state after death as before it was materialled unto life: that the souls of men know neither contrary nor corruption; that they subsist beyond the body, and outlive death by the privilege of their proper natures, and without a miracle: that the souls of the faithful, as they leave earth, take possession of heaven; that those apparitions and ghosts of departed persons are not the wandering souls of men, but the unquiet walks of devils, prompting and suggesting us unto mischief, blood, and villany; instilling and stealing into our hearts that the blessed spirits are not at rest in their graves, but wander, solicitous of the affairs of the world. But that those phantasms appear often, and do frequent cemeteries, charnel-houses, and churches, it is because those are the dormitories of the dead, where the devil, like an insolent champion, beholds with pride the spoils and trophies of his victory over Adam.

§38. — This is that dismal conquest we all deplore, that makes us so often cry, O Adam, *quid fecisti?* I thank God I have not those strait ligaments, or narrow obligations to the world, as to dote on life, or be convulsed and tremble at the name of death. Not that I am insensible of the dread and horror thereof; or, by raking into the bowels of the deceased, continual sight of anatomies, skeletons, or cadaverous relicks, like vespilloes, or gravemakers, I am become stupid, or have forgot the apprehension of mortality; but that, marshalling all the horrors, and contemplating the extremities thereof, I find not anything therein able to daunt the courage of a man, much less a well-resolved Christian; and therefore am not angry at the error of our first parents, or unwilling to bear a part of this common fate, and, like the best of them, to die; that is, to cease to breathe, to take a farewell of the elements; to be a kind of nothing for a moment; to be within one instant of a spirit. When I take a full view and circle of myself without this reasonable moderator, and equal piece of justice, death, I do conceive myself the miserablest person extant. Were there not another life that I hope for, all the vanities of this world should not entreat a moment's breath from me. Could the devil work my belief to imagine I could never die, I would not outlive that very thought. I have so abject a

35

conceit of this common way of existence, this retaining to the sun and elements, I cannot think this is to be a man, or to live according to the dignity of humanity. In expectation of a better, I can with patience embrace this life; yet, in my best meditations, do often defy death. I honour any man that contemns it; nor can I highly love any that is afraid of it: this makes me naturally love a soldier, and honour those tattered and contemptible regiments, that will die at the command of a sergeant. For a pagan there may be some motives to be in love with life; but, for a Christian to be amazed at death, I see not how he can escape this dilemma — that he is too sensible of this life, or hopeless of the life to come.

§39. — Some divines[52] count Adam thirty years old at his creation, because they suppose him created in the perfect age and stature of man: and surely we are all out of the computation of our age; and every man is some months older than he bethinks him; for we live, move, have a being, and are subject to the actions of the elements, and the malice of diseases, in that other world, the truest microcosm, the womb of our mother; for besides that general and common existence we are conceived to hold in our chaos, and whilst we sleep within the bosom of our causes, we enjoy a being and life in three distinct worlds, wherein we receive most manifest gradations. In that obscure world, the womb of our mother, our time is short, computed by the moon; yet longer than the days of many creatures that behold the sun; ourselves being not yet without life, sense, and reason;[53] though, for the manifestation of its actions, it awaits the opportunity of objects, and seems to live there but in its root and soul of vegetation. Entering afterwards upon the scene of the world, we arise up and become another creature; performing the reasonable actions of man, and obscurely manifesting that part of divinity in us, but not in complement and perfection, till we have once more cast our secundine, that is, this slough of flesh, and are delivered into the last world, that is, that ineffable place of Paul, that proper *ubi* of spirits. The smattering I have of the philosopher's stone (which is something more than the perfect exaltation[54] of gold) hath taught me a great deal of divinity, and instructed my belief, how that immortal spirit and incorruptible substance of my soul may lie obscure, and sleep a while within this house of flesh. Those strange and mystical transmigrations that I have observed in silkworms turned my philosophy into divinity. There is in these works of nature, which seem to puzzle reason, something divine; and hath more in it than the eye of a common spectator doth discover.

§40. — I am naturally bashful; nor hath conversation, age, or travel, been able to effront or enharden me; yet I have one part of modesty, which I have seldom discovered in another, that is (to speak truly), I am not so much afraid of death as ashamed thereof; 'tis the very disgrace and ignominy of our natures, that in a moment can so disfigure us, that our nearest friends, wife, and children, stand afraid, and start at us. The birds and beasts of the field, that before, in a natural fear, obeyed us, forgetting all allegiance, begin to prey upon us. This very conceit hath, in a tempest, disposed and left me willing to be swallowed up in the abyss of waters, wherein I had perished unseen, unpitied, without wondering eyes, tears of pity, lectures of mortality, and none had said, "*Quantum mutatus ab illo!*" Not that I am ashamed of the anatomy of my parts, or can accuse nature of playing the bungler in any part of me, or my own vicious life for contracting any shameful disease upon me, whereby I might not call myself as wholesome a morsel for the worms as any.

§41. — Some, upon the courage of a fruitful issue, wherein, as in the truest chronicle, they seem to outlive themselves, can with greater patience away with death. This conceit and counterfeit subsisting in our progenies seems to be a mere fallacy, unworthy the desire of a man, that can but conceive a thought of the next world; who, in a nobler ambition, should desire to live in his substance in heaven, rather than his name and shadow * Who willed his friend not to bury him, but to hang him up with a staff in his hand, to fright away the crows. in the earth. And therefore, at my death, I mean to take a total adieu of the world, not caring for a monument, history, or epitaph; not so much as the bare memory of my name to be found anywhere, but in the universal register of God. I am not yet so cynical, as to approve the testament of Diogenes,* nor do I altogether allow that rodomontado of Lucan;* * "Pharsalia," vii. 819.

——"Coelo tegitur, qui non habet urnam."

He that unburied lies wants not his hearse;

For unto him a tomb's the universe.

but commend, in my calmer judgment, those ingenuous intentions that desire to sleep by the urns of their fathers, and strive to go the neatest way unto corruption. I do not envy the temper[55] of crows and daws, nor the numerous and weary days of our fathers before the flood. If there be any truth in astrology, I may outlive a jubilee;[56] as yet I have not seen one revolution of Saturn,[57] nor hath my pulse beat thirty years, and yet, excepting one,[58] have seen the ashes of, and left under ground, all the kings of Europe; have been contemporary to three emperors, four grand signiors, and as many popes: methinks I have outlived myself, and begin to be weary of the sun; I have shaken hands with delight in my warm blood and canicular days; I perceive I do anticipate the vices of age; the world to me is but a dream or mock-show, and we all therein but pantaloons and anticks, to my severer contemplations.

§42. — It is not, I confess, an unlawful prayer to desire to surpass the days of our Saviour, or wish to outlive that age wherein he thought fittest to die; yet, if (as divinity affirms) there shall be no grey hairs in heaven, but all shall rise in the perfect state of men, we do but outlive those perfections in this world, to be recalled unto them by a greater miracle in the next, and run on here but to be retrograde hereafter. Were there any hopes to outlive vice, or a point to be superannuated from sin, it were worthy our knees to implore the days of Methuselah. But age doth not rectify, but incurvate our natures, turning bad dispositions into worser habits, and (like diseases) brings on incurable vices; for every day, as we grow weaker in age, we grow stronger in sin, and the number of our days doth but make our sins innumerable. The same vice, committed at sixteen, is not the same, though it agrees in all other circumstances, as at forty; but swells and doubles from the circumstance of our ages, wherein, besides the constant and inexcusable habit of transgressing, the maturity of our judgment cuts off pretence unto excuse or pardon. Every sin, the oftener it is committed, the more it acquireth in the quality of evil; as it succeeds in time, so it proceeds in degrees of badness; for as they proceed they ever multiply, and, like figures in arithmetick, the last stands for more than all that went before it. And, though I think no man can live well once, but he that could live twice, yet, for my own part, I would not live over my hours past, or begin again the thread of my days; not upon * *Ep.* lib. xxiv. ep. 24. Cicero's ground,* because I have lived them well, but for fear I should live them worse. I find my growing judgment daily instruct me how to be better, but my untamed affections and confirmed vitiosity make me daily do worse. I find in my confirmed age the same sins I discovered in my youth; I committed many then because I was a child; and, because I commit them still, I am yet an infant. Therefore I perceive a man may be twice a child, before the days of dotage; and stand in need of AEson's bath[59] before threescore.

§43. — And truly there goes a deal of providence to produce a man's life unto threescore; there is more required than an able temper for those years: though the radical humour contain in it sufficient oil for seventy, yet I perceive in some it gives no light past thirty: men assign not all the causes of long life, that write whole books thereof. They that found themselves on the radical balsam, or vital sulphur of the parts, determine not why Abel lived not so long as Adam. There is therefore a secret gloom or bottom of our days: 'twas his wisdom to determine them: but his perpetual and waking providence that fulfils and accomplisheth them; wherein the spirits, ourselves, and all the creatures of God, in a secret and disputed way, do execute his will. Let them not therefore complain of immaturity that die about thirty: they fall but like the whole world, whose solid and well-composed substance must not expect the duration and period of its constitution: when all things are completed in it, its age is accomplished; and the last and general fever may as naturally destroy it before six thousand,[60] as me before forty. There is therefore some other hand that twines the thread of life than that of nature: we are not only ignorant in antipathies and occult qualities; our ends are as obscure as our beginnings; the line of our days is drawn by night, and the various effects therein by a pencil that is invisible; wherein, though we confess our ignorance, I am sure we do not err if we say, it is the hand of God.

$44. — I am much taken with two verses of Lucan, since I have been able not only, as we do at school, to construe, but understand:

* *Pharsalia*, iv. 519.

"Victurosque Dei celant ut vivere, durent,

Felix esse mori."*

We're all deluded, vainly searching ways

To make us happy by the length of days;

For cunningly, to make's protract this breath,

The gods conceal the happiness of death.

There be many excellent strains in that poet, wherewith his stoical genius hath liberally supplied him: and truly there are singular pieces in the philosophy of Zeno,[61] and doctrine of the stoics, which I perceive, delivered in a pulpit, pass for current divinity: yet herein are they in extremes, that can allow a man to be his own assassin, and so highly extol the end and suicide of Cato. This is indeed not to fear death, but yet to be afraid of life. It is a brave act of valour to contemn death; but, where life is more terrible than death, it is then the truest valour to dare to live: and herein religion hath taught us a noble example; for all the valiant acts of Curtius, Scaevola, or Codrus, do not parallel, or match, that one of Job; and sure there is no torture to the rack of a disease, nor any poniards in death itself, like those in the way or prologue unto it. "Emori nolo, sed me esse mortuum nihil curo;" I would not die, but care not to be dead. Were I of Caesar's religion,[62] I should be of his desires, and wish rather to go off at one blow, than to be sawed in pieces by the grating torture of a disease. Men that look no further than their outsides, think health an appurtenance unto life, and quarrel with their constitutions for being sick; but I, that have examined the parts of man, and know upon what tender filaments that fabrick hangs, do wonder that we are not always so; and, considering the thousand doors that lead to death, do thank my God that we can die but once. 'Tis not only the mischief of diseases, and the villany of poisons, that make an end of us; we vainly accuse the fury of guns, and the new inventions of death:— it is in the power of every hand to destroy us, and we are beholden unto every one we meet, he doth not kill us. There is therefore but one comfort left, that though it be in the power of the weakest arm to take away life, it is not in the strongest to deprive us of death. God would not exempt himself from that; the misery of immortality in the flesh he undertook not, that was immortal. Certainly there is no happiness within this circle of flesh; nor is it in the opticks of these eyes to behold felicity. The first day of our jubilee is death; the devil hath therefore failed of his desires; we are happier with death than we should have been without it: there is no misery but in himself, where there is no end of misery; and so indeed, in his own sense, the stoic is in the right.[63] He forgets that he can die, who complains of misery: we are in the power of no calamity while death is in our own.

§45. — Now, besides this literal and positive kind of death, there are others whereof divines make mention, and those, I think, not merely metaphorical, as mortification, dying unto sin and the world. Therefore, I say, every man hath a double horoscope; one of his humanity — his birth, another of his Christianity — his baptism: and from this do I compute or calculate my nativity; not reckoning those *horae combustae,*[64] and odd days, or esteeming myself anything, before I was my Saviour's and enrolled in the register of Christ. Whosoever enjoys not this life, I count him but an apparition, though he wear about him the sensible affections of flesh. In these moral acceptions, the way to be immortal is to die daily; nor can I think I have the true theory of death, when I contemplate a skull or behold a skeleton with those vulgar imaginations it casts upon us. I have therefore enlarged that common *memento mori* into a more Christian memorandum, *memento quatuor novissima* — those four inevitable points of us all, death, judgment, heaven, and hell. Neither did the contemplations of the heathens rest in their graves, without a further thought, of Rhadamanth[65] or some judicial proceeding after death, though in another way, and upon suggestion of their natural reasons. I cannot but marvel from what sibyl or oracle they stole the prophecy of the world's destruction by fire, or whence Lucan learned to say —

* *Pharsalia*, vii. 814.

"Communis mundo superest rogus, ossibus astra

Misturus —"*

There yet remains to th' world one common fire,

Wherein our bones with stars shall make one pyre.

I believe the world grows near its end; yet is neither old nor decayed, nor will ever perish upon the ruins of its own principles. As the work of creation was above nature, so its adversary, annihilation; without which the world hath not its end, but its mutation. Now, what force should be able to consume it thus far, without the breath of God, which is the truest consuming flame, my philosophy cannot inform me. Some believe there went not a minute to the world's creation, nor shall there go to its destruction; those six days, so punctually described, make not to them one moment, but rather seem to manifest the method and idea of that great work of the intellect of God than the manner how he proceeded in its operation. I cannot dream that there should be at the last day any such judicial proceeding, or calling to the bar, as indeed the Scripture seems to imply, and the literal commentators do conceive: for unspeakable mysteries in the Scriptures are often delivered in a vulgar and illustrative way, and, being written unto man, are delivered, not as they truly are, but as they may be understood; wherein, notwithstanding, the different interpretations according to different capacities may stand firm with our devotion, nor be any way prejudicial to each single edification.

§46. — Now, to determine the day and year of this inevitable time, is not only convincible and statute madness, but also manifest impiety. How shall we interpret Elias's six thousand years, or imagine the secret communicated to a Rabbi which God hath denied unto his angels? It had been an excellent quaere to have posed the devil of Delphos, and must needs have forced him to some strange amphibology. It hath not only mocked the predictions of sundry astrologers in ages past, but the prophecies of many melancholy heads in these present; who, neither understanding reasonably things past nor present, pretend a knowledge of things to come; heads ordained only to manifest the incredible * "In those days there shall come liars and false prophets." effects of melancholy and to fulfil old prophecies,* rather than be the authors of new. "In those days there shall come wars and rumours of wars" to me seems no prophecy, but a constant truth in all times verified since it was pronounced. "There shall be signs in the moon and stars;" how comes he then like a thief in the night, when he gives an item of his coming? That common sign, drawn from the revelation of antichrist, is as obscure as any; in our common compute he hath been come these many years; but, for my own part, to speak freely, I am half of opinion that antichrist is the philosopher's stone in divinity, for the discovery and invention whereof, though there be prescribed rules, and probable inductions, yet hath hardly any man attained the perfect discovery thereof. That general opinion, that the world grows near its end, hath possessed all ages past as nearly as ours. I am afraid that the souls that now depart cannot escape that lingering expostulation of the saints under the altar, "quousque, Domine?" how long, O Lord? and groan in the expectation of the great jubilee.

§47. — This is the day that must make good that great attribute of God, his justice; that must reconcile those unanswerable doubts that torment the wisest understandings; and reduce those seeming inequalities and respective distributions in this world, to an equality and recompensive justice in the next. This is that one day, that shall include and comprehend all that went before it; wherein, as in the last scene, all the actors must enter, to complete and make up the catastrophe of this great piece. This is the day whose memory hath, only, power to make us honest in the dark, and to be virtuous without a witness. "Ipsa sui pretium virtus sibi," that virtue is her own reward, is but a cold principle, and not able to maintain our variable resolutions in a constant and settled way of goodness. I have practised that honest artifice of Seneca,⁶⁶ and, in my retired and solitary imaginations to detain me from the foulness of vice, have fancied to myself the presence of my dear and worthiest friends, before whom I should lose my head rather than be vicious; yet herein I found that there was nought but moral honesty; and this was not to be virtuous for his sake who must reward us at the last. I have tried if I could reach that great resolution of his, to be honest without a thought of heaven or hell; and, indeed I found, upon a natural inclination, and inbred loyalty unto virtue, that I could serve her without a livery, yet not in that resolved and venerable way, but that the frailty of my nature, upon an easy temptation, might be induced to forget her. The life, therefore, and spirit of all our actions is the resurrection, and a stable apprehension that our ashes shall enjoy the fruit of our pious endeavours; without this, all religion is a fallacy, and those impieties of Lucian, Euripides, and Julian, are no blasphemies, but subtile verities; and atheists have been the only philosophers.

§48. — How shall the dead arise, is no question of my faith; to believe only possibilities is not faith, but mere philosophy. Many things are true in divinity, which are neither inducible by reason nor confirmable by sense; and many things in philosophy confirmable by sense, yet not inducible by reason. Thus it is impossible, by any solid or demonstrative reasons, to persuade a man to believe the conversion of the needle to the north; though this be possible and true, and easily credible, upon a single experiment unto the sense. I believe that our estranged and divided ashes shall unite again; that our separated dust, after so many pilgrimages and transformations into the parts of minerals, plants, animals, elements, shall, at the voice of God, return into their primitive shapes, and join again to make up their primary and predestinate forms. As at the creation there was a separation of that confused mass into its pieces; so at the destruction thereof there shall be a separation into its distinct individuals. As, at the creation of the world, all the distinct species that we behold lay involved in one mass, till the fruitful voice of God separated this united multitude into its several species, so, at the last day, when those corrupted relicks shall be scattered in the wilderness of forms, and seem to have forgot their proper habits, God, by a powerful voice, shall command them back into their proper shapes, and call them out by their single individuals. Then shall appear the fertility of Adam, and the magick of that sperm that hath dilated into so many millions. I have often beheld, as a miracle, that artificial resurrection and revivification of mercury, how being mortified into a thousand shapes, it assumes again its own, and returns into its numerical self. Let us speak naturally, and like philosophers. The forms of alterable bodies in these sensible corruptions perish not; nor, as we imagine, wholly quit their mansions; but retire and contract themselves into their secret and unaccessible parts; where they may best protect themselves from the action of their antagonist. A plant or vegetable consumed to ashes to a contemplative and school-philosopher seems utterly destroyed, and the form to have taken his leave for ever; but to a sensible artist the forms are not perished, but withdrawn into their incombustible part, where they lie secure from the action of that devouring element. This is made good by experience, which can from the ashes of a plant revive the plant, and from its cinders recall it into its stalk and leaves again.[67] What the art of man can do in these inferior pieces, what blasphemy is it to affirm the finger of God cannot do in those more perfect and sensible structures? This is that mystical philosophy, from whence no true scholar becomes an atheist, but from the visible effects of nature grows up a real divine, and beholds not in a dream, as Ezekiel, but in an ocular and visible object, the types of his resurrection.

§49. — Now, the necessary mansions of our restored selves are those two contrary and incompatible places we call heaven and hell. To define them, or strictly to determine what and where these are, surpasseth my divinity. That elegant apostle, which seemed to have a glimpse of heaven, hath left but a negative description thereof; which "neither eye hath seen, nor ear hath heard, nor can enter into the heart of man:" he was translated out of himself to behold it; but, being returned into himself, could not express it. Saint John's description by emeralds, chrysolites, and precious stones, is too weak to express the material heaven we behold. Briefly, therefore, where the soul hath the full measure and complement of happiness; where the boundless appetite of that spirit remains completely satisfied that it can neither desire addition nor alteration; that, I think, is truly heaven: and this can only be in the enjoyment of that essence, whose infinite goodness is able to terminate the desires of itself, and the unsatiable wishes of ours. Wherever God will thus manifest himself, there is heaven, though within the circle of this sensible world. Thus, the soul of man may be in heaven anywhere, even within the limits of his own proper body; and when it ceaseth to live in the body it may remain in its own soul, that is, its Creator. And thus we may say that Saint Paul, whether in the body or out of the body, was yet in heaven. To place it in the empyreal, or beyond the tenth sphere, is to forget the world's destruction; for when this sensible world shall be destroyed, all shall then be here as it is now there, an empyreal heaven, a *quasi* vacuity; when to ask where heaven is, is to demand where the presence of God is, or where we have the glory of that happy vision. Moses, that was bred up in all the learning of the Egyptians, committed a gross absurdity in philosophy, when with these eyes of flesh he desired to see God, and petitioned his Maker, that is truth itself, to a contradiction. Those that imagine heaven and hell neighbours, and conceive a vicinity between those two extremes, upon consequence of the parable, where Dives discoursed with Lazarus, in Abraham's bosom, do too grossly conceive of those glorified creatures, whose eyes shall easily out-see the sun, and behold without perspective the extremest distances: for if there shall be, in our glorified eyes, the faculty of sight and reception of objects, I could think the visible species there to be in as unlimitable a way as now the intellectual. I grant that two bodies placed beyond the tenth sphere, or in a vacuity, according to Aristotle's philosophy, could not behold each other, because there wants a body or medium to hand and transport the visible rays of the object unto the sense; but when there shall be a general defect of either medium to convey, or light to prepare and dispose that medium, and yet a perfect vision, we must suspend the rules of our philosophy, and make all good by a more absolute piece of opticks.

§50. — I cannot tell how to say that fire is the essence of hell; I know not what to make of purgatory, or conceive a flame that can either prey upon, or purify the substance of a soul. Those flames of sulphur, mentioned in the scriptures, I take not to be understood of this present hell, but of that to come, where fire shall make up the complement of our tortures, and have a body or subject whereon to manifest its tyranny. Some who have had the honour to be textuary in divinity are of opinion it shall be the same specifical fire with ours. This is hard to conceive, yet can I make good how even that may prey upon our bodies, and yet not consume us: for in this material world, there are bodies that persist invincible in the powerfulest flames; and though, by the action of fire, they fall into ignition and liquation, yet will they never suffer a destruction. I would gladly know how Moses, with an actual fire, calcined or burnt the golden calf into powder: for that mystical metal of gold, whose solary and celestial nature I admire, exposed unto the violence of fire, grows only hot, and liquefies, but consumeth not; so when the consumable and volatile pieces of our bodies shall be refined into a more impregnable and fixed temper, like gold, though they suffer from the action of flames, they shall never perish, but lie immortal in the arms of fire. And surely, if this flame must suffer only by the action of this element, there will many bodies escape; and not only heaven, but earth will not be at an end, but rather a beginning. For at present it is not earth, but a composition of fire, water, earth, and air; but at that time, spoiled of these ingredients, it shall appear in a substance more like itself, its ashes. Philosophers that opinioned the world's destruction by fire, did never dream of annihilation, which is beyond the power of sublunary causes; for the last and proper action of that element is but vitrification, or a reduction of a body into glass; and therefore some of our chymicks facetiously affirm, that, at the last fire, all shall be crystalized and reverberated into glass, which is the utmost action of that element. Nor need we fear this term, annihilation, or wonder that God will destroy the works of his creation: for man subsisting, who is, and will then truly appear, a microcosm, the world cannot be said to be destroyed. For the eyes of God, and perhaps also of our glorified selves, shall as really behold and contemplate the world, in its epitome or contracted essence, as now it doth at large and in its dilated substance. In the seed of a plant, to the eyes of God, and to the understanding of man, there exists, though in an invisible way, the perfect leaves, flowers, and fruit thereof; for things that are in *posse* to the sense, are actually existent to the understanding. Thus God beholds all things, who contemplates as fully his works in their epitome as in their full volume, and beheld as amply the whole world, in that little compendium of the sixth day, as in the scattered and dilated pieces of those five before.

§51. — Men commonly set forth the torments of hell by fire, and the extremity of corporal afflictions, and describe hell in the same method that Mahomet doth heaven. This indeed makes a noise, and drums in popular ears: but if this be the terrible piece thereof, it is not worthy to stand in diameter with heaven, whose happiness consists in that part that is best able to comprehend it, that immortal essence, that translated divinity and colony of God, the soul. Surely, though we place hell under earth, the devil's walk and purlieu is about it. Men speak too popularly who place it in those flaming mountains, which to grosser apprehensions represent hell. The heart of man is the place the devils dwell in; I feel sometimes a hell within myself; Lucifer keeps his court in my breast; Legion is revived in me. There are as many hells as Anaxagoras[68] conceited worlds. There was more than one hell in Magdalene, when there were seven devils; for every devil is an hell unto himself,[69] he holds enough of torture in his own *ubi*; and needs not the misery of circumference to afflict him: and thus, a distracted con science here is a shadow or introduction unto hell hereafter. Who can but pity the merciful intention of those hands that do destroy themselves? The devil, were it in his power, would do the like; which being impossible, his miseries are endless, and he suffers most in that attribute wherein he is impassible, his immortality.

§52. — I thank God, and with joy I mention it, I was never afraid of hell, nor ever grew pale at the description of that place. I have so fixed my contemplations on heaven, that I have almost forgot the idea of hell; and am afraid rather to lose the joys of the one, than endure the misery of the other: to be deprived of them is a perfect hell, and needs methinks no addition to complete our afflictions. That terrible term hath never detained me from sin, nor do I owe any good action to the name thereof. I fear God, yet am not afraid of him; his mercies make me ashamed of my sins, before his judgments afraid thereof: these are the forced and secondary method of his wisdom, which he useth but as the last remedy, and upon provocation; — a course rather to deter the wicked, than incite the virtuous to his worship. I can hardly think there was ever any scared into heaven: they go the fairest way to heaven that would serve God without a hell: other mercenaries, that crouch unto him in fear of hell, though they term themselves the servants, are indeed but the slaves, of the Almighty.

§53. — And to be true, and speak my soul, when I survey the occurrences of my life, and call into account the finger of God, I can perceive nothing but an abyss and mass of mercies, either in general to mankind, or in particular to myself. And, whether out of the prejudice of my affection, or an inverting and partial conceit of his mercies, I know not — but those which others term crosses, afflictions, judgments, misfortunes, to me, who inquire further into them than their visible effects, they both appear, and in event have ever proved, the secret and dissembled favours of his affection. It is a singular piece of wisdom to apprehend truly, and without passion, the works of God, and so well to distinguish his justice from his mercy as not to miscall those noble attributes; yet it is likewise an honest piece of logick so to dispute and argue the proceedings of God as to distinguish even his judgments into mercies. For God is merciful unto all, because better to the worst than the best deserve; and to say he punisheth none in this world, though it be a paradox, is no absurdity. To one that hath committed murder, if the judge should only ordain a fine, it were a madness to call this a punishment, and to repine at the sentence, rather than admire the clemency of the judge. Thus, our offences being mortal, and deserving not only death but damnation, if the goodness of God be content to traverse and pass them over with a loss, misfortune, or disease; what frenzy were it to term this a punishment, rather than an extremity of mercy, and to groan under the rod of his judgments rather than admire the sceptre of his mercies! Therefore to adore, honour, and admire him, is a debt of gratitude due from the obligation of our nature, states, and conditions: and with these thoughts he that knows them best will not deny that I adore him. That I obtain heaven, and the bliss thereof, is accidental, and not the intended work of my devotion; it being a felicity I can neither think to deserve nor scarce in modesty to expect. For these two ends of us all, either as rewards or punishments, are mercifully ordained and disproportionably disposed unto our actions; the one being so far beyond our deserts, the other so infinitely below our demerits.

§54. — There is no salvation to those that believe not in Christ; that is, say some, since his nativity, and, as divinity affirmeth, before also; which makes me much apprehend the end of those honest worthies and philosophers which died before his incarnation. It is hard to place those souls in hell, whose worthy lives do teach us virtue on earth. Methinks, among those many subdivisions of hell, there might have been one limbo left for these. What a strange vision will it be to see their poetical fictions converted into verities, and their imagined and fancied furies into real devils! How strange to them will sound the history of Adam, when they shall suffer for him they never heard of! When they who derive their genealogy from the gods, shall know they are the unhappy issue of sinful man! It is an insolent part of reason, to controvert the works of God, or question the justice of his proceedings. Could humility teach others, as it hath instructed me, to contemplate the infinite and incomprehensible distance betwixt the Creator and the creature; or did we seriously perpend that one simile of St Paul, "shall the vessel say to the potter, why hast thou made me thus?" it would prevent these arrogant disputes of reason: nor would we argue the definitive sentence of God, either to heaven or hell. Men that live according to the right rule and law of reason, live but in their own kind, as beasts do in theirs; who justly obey the prescript of their natures, and therefore cannot reasonably demand a reward of their actions, as only obeying the natural dictates of their reason. It will, therefore, and must, at last appear, that all salvation is through Christ; which verity, I fear, these great examples of virtue must confirm, and make it good how the perfectest actions of earth have no title or claim unto heaven.

§55. — Nor truly do I think the lives of these, or of any other, were ever correspondent, or in all points conformable, unto their doctrines. It is evident that Aristotle transgressed the rule of his own ethicks;[70] the stoicks, that condemn passion, and command a man to laugh in Phalaris's[71] bull, could not endure without a groan a fit of the stone or colick. The scepticks, that affirmed they knew nothing,[72] even in that opinion confute themselves, and thought they knew more than all the world beside. Diogenes I hold to be the most vain-glorious man of his time, and more ambitious in refusing all honours, than Alexander in rejecting none. Vice and the devil put a fallacy upon our reasons; and, provoking us too hastily to run from it, entangle and profound us deeper in it. The duke of Venice, that weds himself unto the sea, by a ring of gold,[73] I will not accuse of prodigality, because it is a solemnity of good use and consequence in the state: but the philosopher, that threw his money into the sea to avoid avarice, was a notorious prodigal.[74] There is no road or ready way to virtue; it is not an easy point of art to disentangle ourselves from this riddle or web of sin. To perfect virtue, as to religion, there is required a *panoplia*, or complete armour; that whilst we lie at close ward against one vice, we lie not open to the veney[75] of another. And indeed wiser discretions, that have the thread of reason to conduct them, offend without a pardon; whereas under heads may stumble without dishonour. There go so many circumstances to piece up one good action, that it is a lesson to be good, and we are forced to be virtuous by the book. Again, the practice of men holds not an equal pace, yea and often runs counter to their theory; we naturally know what is good, but naturally pursue what is evil: the rhetorick wherewith I persuade another cannot persuade myself. There is a depraved appetite in us, that will with patience hear the learned instructions of reason, but yet perform no further than agrees to its own irregular humour. In brief, we all are monsters; that is, a composition of man and beast: wherein we must endeavour to be as the poets fancy that wise man, Chiron; that is, to have the region of man above that of beast, and sense to sit but at the feet of reason. Lastly, I do desire with God that all, but yet affirm with men that few, shall know salvation — that the bridge is narrow, the passage strait unto life: yet those who do confine the church of God either to particular nations, churches, or families, have made it far narrower than our Saviour ever meant it.

§56. — The vulgarity of those judgments that wrap the church of God in Strabo's cloak,[76] and restrain it unto Europe, seem to me as bad geographers as Alexander, who thought he had conquered all the world, when he had not subdued the half of any part thereof. For we cannot deny the church of God both in Asia and Africa, if we do not forget the peregrinations of the apostles, the deaths of the martyrs, the sessions of many and (even in our reformed judgment) lawful councils, held in those parts in the minority and nonage of ours. Nor must a few differences, more remarkable in the eyes of man than, perhaps, in the judgment of God, excommunicate from heaven one another; much less those Christians who are in a manner all martyrs, maintaining their faith in the noble way of persecution, and serving God in the fire, whereas we honour him in the sunshine.

'Tis true, we all hold there is a number of elect, and many to be saved; yet, take our opinions together, and from the confusion thereof, there will be no such thing as salvation, nor shall any one be saved: for, first, the church of Rome condemneth us; we likewise them; the subreformists and sectaries sentence the doctrine of our church as damnable; the atomist, or familist,[77] reprobates all these; and all these, them again. Thus, whilst the mercies of God do promise us heaven, our conceits and opinions exclude us from that place. There must be therefore more than one St Peter;

particular churches and sects usurp the gates of heaven, and turn the key against each other; and thus we go to heaven against each other's wills, conceits, and opinions, and, with as much uncharity as ignorance, do err, I fear, in points not only of our own, but one another's salvation.

§57. — I believe many are saved who to man seem reprobated, and many are reprobated who in the opinion and sentence of man stand elected. There will appear, at the last day, strange and unexpected examples, both of his justice and his mercy; and, therefore, to define either is folly in man, and insolency even in the devils. These acute and subtile spirits, in all their sagacity, can hardly divine who shall be saved; which if they could prognostick, their labour were at an end, nor need they compass the earth, seeking whom they may devour. Those who, upon a rigid application of the law, sentence Solomon unto damnation,[78] condemn not only him, but themselves, and the whole world; for by the letter and written word of God, we are without exception in the state of death: but there is a prerogative of God, and an arbitrary pleasure above the letter of his own law, by which alone we can pretend unto salvation, and through which Solomon might be as easily saved as those who condemn him.

§58. — The number of those who pretend unto salvation, and those infinite swarms who think to pass through the eye of this needle, have much amazed me. That name and compellation of "little flock" doth not comfort, but deject, my devotion; especially when I reflect upon mine own unworthiness, wherein, according to my humble apprehensions, I am below them all. I believe there shall never be an anarchy in heaven; but, as there are hierarchies amongst the angels, so shall there be degrees of priority amongst the saints. Yet is it, I protest, beyond my ambition to aspire unto the first ranks; my desires only are, and I shall be happy therein, to be but the last man, and bring up the rear in heaven.

§59. — Again, I am confident, and fully persuaded, yet dare not take my oath, of my salvation. I am, as it were, sure, and do believe without all doubt, that there is such a city as Constantinople; yet, for me to take my oath thereon were a kind of perjury, because I hold no infallible warrant from my own sense to confirm me in the certainty thereof. And truly, though many pretend to an absolute certainty of their salvation, yet when an humble soul shall contemplate our own unworthiness, she shall meet with many doubts, and suddenly find how little we stand in need of the precept of St Paul, "work out your salvation *with fear and trembling*." That which is the cause of my election, I hold to be the cause of my salvation, which was the mercy and *beneplacit* of God, before I was, or the foundation of the world. "Before Abraham was, I am," is the saying of Christ, yet is it true in some sense if I say it of myself; for I was not only before myself but Adam, that is, in the idea of God, and the decree of that synod held from all eternity. And in this sense, I say, the world was before the creation, and at an end before it had a beginning. And thus was I dead before I was alive; though my grave be England, my dying place was Paradise; and Eve miscarried of me, before she conceived of Cain.

$60. — Insolent zeals, that do decry good works and rely only upon faith, take not away merit: for, depending upon the efficacy of their faith, they enforce the condition of God, and in a more sophistical way do seem to challenge heaven. It was decreed by God that only those that lapped in the water like dogs, should have the honour to destroy the Midianites; yet could none of those justly challenge, or imagine he deserved, that honour thereupon. I do not deny but that true faith, and such as God requires, is not only a mark or token, but also a means, of our salvation; but, where to find this, is as obscure to me as my last end. And if our Saviour could object, unto his own disciples and favourites, a faith that, to the quantity of a grain of mustard seed, is able to remove mountains; surely that which we boast of is not anything, or, at the most, but a remove from nothing.

This is the tenour of my belief; wherein, though there be many things singular, and to the humour of my irregular self, yet, if they square not with maturer judgments, I disclaim them, and do no further favour them than the learned and best judgments shall authorize them.

[1]. It was a proverb, "Ubi tres medici duo athei."

[2]. A Latinised word meaning a taunt (impropero.)

[3]. The synod of Dort was held in 1619 to discuss the doctrines of Arminius. It ended by condemning them.

[4]. Hallam, commenting on this passage, says —"That Jesuit must be a disgrace to his order who would have asked more than such a concession to secure a proselyte — the right of interpreting whatever was written, and of supplying whatever was not"— *Hist. England*, vol. ii. p. 74.

[5]. See the statute of the Six Articles (31 Hen. VIII. c. 14), which declared that transubstantiation, communion in one kind, celibacy of the clergy,

vows of widowhood, private masses, and auricular confession, were part of the law of England.

6. In the year 1606, when the Jesuits were expelled from Venice, Pope Paul V. threatened to excommunicate that republic. A most violent quarrel ensued, which was ultimately settled by the mediation of France.

7. Alluding to the story of OEdipus solving the riddle proposed by the Sphynx.

8. The nymph Arethusa was changed by Diana into a fountain, and was said to have flowed under the sea from Elis to the fountain of Arethusa near Syracuse. — Ov. *Met.* lib. v. fab. 8.

9. These heretics denied the immortality of the soul, but held that it was recalled to life with the body. Origen came from Egypt to confute them, and is said to have succeeded. (See Mosh. *Eccl. Hist.*, lib. i. c. 5. sec. 16.) Pope John XXII. afterwards adopted it.

10. A division from the Greek [Greek omitted].

11. The brain.

12. A faint resemblance, from the Latin *adumbro*, to shade.

13. Alluding to the idea Sir T. Browne often expresses, that an oracle was the utterance of the devil.

14. To fathom, from Latin *profundis*.

15. Beginning from the Latin *efficio*.

16. Galen's great work.

17. John de Monte Regio made a wooden eagle that, when the emperor was entering Nuremburg, flew to meet him, and hovered over his head. He also made an iron fly that, when at dinner, he was able to make start from under his hand, and fly round the table. — See De Bartas, 6me jour 1me semaine.

18. Hidden, from the Greek [Greek omitted].

[19]. A military term for a small mine.

[20]. The Armada.

[21]. The practice of drawing lots.

[22]. An account.

[23]. See Il. VIII. 18 —

"Let down our golden everlasting chain,

Whose strong embrace holds heaven, and earth, and main."

— *Pope*, Il. viii. 26.

[24]. An argument where one proposition is accumulated upon another, from the Greek [Greek omitted], a heap.

[25]. Alluding to the second triumvirate — that of Augustus, Antony, and Lepidus. Florus says of it, "Respublica convulsa est lacerataque."

[26]. Ochinus. He was first a monk, then a doctor, then a Capuchin friar, then a Protestant: in 1547 he came to England, and was very active in the Reformation. He was afterwards made Canon of Canterbury. The Socinians claim him as one of their sect.

[27]. The father of Pantagruel. His adventures are given in the first book of Rabelais, Sir Bevys of Hampton, a metrical romance, relating the adventures of Sir Bevys with the saracens. — Wright and Halliwell's *Reliquiae Antiquae*, ii. 59.

[28]. Contradictions between two laws.

[29]. On his arrival at Paris, Pantagruel visited the library of St. Victor: he states a list of the works he found there, among which was "Tartaretus." Pierre Tartaret was a French doctor who disputed with Duns Scotus. His works were republished at Lyons, 1621.

[30]. Deucalion was king of Thessaly at the time of the deluge. He and his wife Pyrrha, with the advice of the oracle of Themis, repeopled the earth

by throwing behind them the bones of their grand-mother — *i.e.*, stones of the earth. — See Ovid, *Met.* lib. i. fab. 7.

[31]. St. Augustine (De Civ. Dei, xvi. 7).

[32]. [Greek omitted] (St. Matt. xxvii. 5) means death by choking. Erasmus translates it, "abiens laqueo se suspendit."

[33]. Burnt by order of the Caliph Omar, A.D. 640. It contained 700,000 volumes, which served the city for fuel instead of wood for six months.

[34]. Enoch being informed by Adam the world was to be drowned and burnt, made two pillars, one of stone to withstand the water, and one of brick to withstand the fire, and inscribed upon them all known knowledge. — See Josephus, *Ant. Jud.*

[35]. A Franciscan friar, counsellor to the Inquisition, who visited the principal libraries in Spain to make a catalogue of the books opposed to the Romish religion. His "index novus librorum prohibitorum" was published at Seville in 1631.

[36]. Printing, gunpowder, clocks.

[37]. The Targums and the various Talmuds.

[38]. Pagans, Mahometans, Jews, Christians.

[39]. Valour, and death in battle.

[40]. Held 1414–1418.

[41]. Vergilius, bishop of Salzburg, having asserted the existence of Antipodes, the Archbishop of Metz declared him to be a heretic, and caused him to be burnt.

[42]. On searching on Mount Calvary for the true cross, the empress found three. As she was uncertain which was the right one, she caused them to be applied to the body of a dead man, and the one that restored him to life was determined to be the true cross.

[43]. The critical time in human life.

[44]. Oracles were said to have ceased when Christ came, the reply to Augustus on the subject being the last —

"Me puer Hebraeus divos Deus ipse gubernans

Cedere sede jubet tristemque redire sub Orcum

Aris ergo de hinc tacitus discedito nostris."

[45]. An historian who wrote "De Rebus Indicis." He is cited by Pliny, Strabo, and Josephus.

[46]. Alluding to the popular superstition that infant children were carried off by fairies, and others left in their places.

[47]. Who is said to have lived without meat, on the smell of a rose.

[48]. "Essentiae rationalis immortalis."

[49]. St. Augustine, De Civ. Dei, lib. x., cc. 9, 19, 32.

[50]. That which includes everything is opposed to nullity.

[51]. An inversion of the parts of an antithesis.

[52]. St. Augustine —"Homily on Genesis."

[53]. Sir T. Browne wrote a dialogue between two twins in the womb respecting the world into which they were going!

[54]. Refinement.

[55]. Constitution another form of temperament.

[56]. The Jewish computation for fifty years.

[57]. Saturn revolves once in thirty years.

[58]. Christian IV., of Denmark, who reigned from 1588–1647.

59. AEson was the father of Jason. By bathing in a bath prepared for him by Medaea with some magic spells, he became young again. Ovid describes the bath and its ingredients, *Met.*, lib. vii. fab. 2.

60. Alluding to the rabbinical tradition that the world would last for 6000 years, attributed to Elias, and cited in the Talmud.

61. Zeno was the founder of the Stoics.

62. Referring to a passage in Suetonius, Vit. J. Caesar, sec 87:—

"Aspernatus tam lentum mortis genus subitam sibi celeremque optaverat."

63. In holding

"Mors ultima poena est,

Nec metuenda viris."

64. The period when the moon is in conjunction and obscured by the sun.

65. One of the judges of hell.

66. To select some great man for our ideal, and always to act as if he was present with us. See Seneca, lib. i. Ep. 11.

67. Sir T. Browne seems to have made various experiments in this subject. D'Israeli refers to it in his "Curiosities of Literature." Dr Power, a friend of Sir T. Browne, with whom he corresponded, fives a receipt for the process.

68. The celebrated Greek philosopher who taught that the sun was a mass of heated stone, and various other astronomical doctrines. Some critics say Anaxarchus is meant here.

69. See Milton's "Paradise Lost," lib. I. 254 —

"The mind is its own place, and in itself

Can make a heaven of hell, a hell of heaven."

And also Lucretius —

"Hic Acherusia fit stultorum denique vita."— iii. 1023.

[70]. Keck says here —"So did they all, as Lactantius has observed at large. Aristotle is said to have been guilty of great vanity in his clothes, of incontinency, and of unfaithfulness to his master, Alexander II."

[71]. Phalaris, king of Agrigentum, who, when Perillus made a brazen bull in which to kill criminals, placed him in it to try its effects.

[72]. Their maxim was

"Nihil sciri siquis putat id quoque nescit,

An sciri possit quod se nil scire fatetur."

[73]. Pope Alexander III., in his declaration to the Doge, said — "Que la mer vous soit soumise comme l'epouse l'est a son epoux puisque vous in avez acquis l'empire par la victorie." In commemoration of this the Doge and Senate went yearly to Lio, and throwing a ring into the water, claimed the sea as their bride.

[74]. Appolonius Thyaneus, who threw a large quantity of gold into the sea, saying, "Pessundo divitias ne pessundare ab illis."

[75]. The technical term in fencing for a hit —

"A sweet touch, a quick venew of wit."

Love's Labour Lost, act v. sc. 1.

[76]. Strabo compared the configuration of the world, as then known, to a cloak or mantle (*chlamys*).

[77]. Atomists or familists were a Puritanical sect who appeared about 1575, founded by Henry Nicholas, a Dutchman. They considered that the doctrine of revelation was an allegory, and believed that they had attained to spiritual perfection. — See Neal's Hist. of Puritans, 1. 273.

[78]. From the 126th psalm St Augustine contends that Solomon is damned. See also Lyra in 2 Kings vii.

Part the Second

Now, for that other virtue of charity, without which faith is a mere notion and of no existence, I have ever endeavoured to nourish the merciful disposition and humane inclination I borrowed from my parents, and regulate it to the written and prescribed laws of charity. And, if I hold the true anatomy of myself, I am delineated and naturally framed to such a piece of virtue — for I am of a constitution so general that it consorts and sympathizeth with all things; I have no antipathy, or rather idiosyncrasy, in diet, humour, air, anything. I wonder not at the French for their dishes of frogs, snails, and toadstools, nor at the Jews for locusts and grasshoppers; but, being amongst them, make them my common viands; and I find they agree with my stomach as well as theirs. I could digest a salad gathered in a church-yard as well as in a garden. I cannot start at the presence of a serpent, scorpion, lizard, or salamander; at the sight of a toad or viper, I find in me no desire to take up a stone to destroy them. I feel not in myself those common antipathies that I can discover in others: those national repugnances do not touch me, nor do I behold with prejudice the French, Italian, Spaniard, or Dutch; but, where I find their actions in balance with my countrymen's, I honour, love, and embrace them, in the same degree. I was born in the eighth climate, but seem to be framed and constellated unto all. I am no plant that will not prosper out of a garden. All places, all airs, make unto me one country; I am in England everywhere, and under any meridian. I have been shipwrecked, yet am not enemy with the sea or winds; I can study, play, or sleep, in a tempest. In brief I am averse from nothing: my conscience would give me the lie if I should say I absolutely detest or hate any essence, but the devil; or so at least abhor anything, but that we might come to composition. If there be any among those common objects of hatred I do contemn and laugh at, it is that great enemy of reason, virtue, and religion, the multitude; that numerous piece of monstrosity, which, taken asunder, seem men, and the reasonable creatures of God, but, confused together, make but one great beast, and a monstrosity more prodigious than Hydra. It is no breach of charity to call these fools; it is the style all holy writers have afforded them, set down by Solomon in canonical Scripture, and a point of our faith to believe so. Neither in the name of multitude do I only include the base and minor sort of people: there is a rabble even amongst the gentry; a sort of plebeian heads, whose fancy moves with the same wheel as these; men in the same level with mechanicks, though their fortunes do somewhat gild their infirmities, and their purses compound for their follies. But, as in casting account three or four men together come short in account of one man placed by himself below them, so neither are a troop of these ignorant Doradoes[79] of that true esteem and value as many a forlorn person, whose condition doth place him below their feet. Let us speak like politicians; there is a nobility without heraldry, a natural dignity, whereby one man is ranked with another, another filed before him, according to the quality of his desert, and preeminence of his good parts. Though the corruption of these times, and the bias of present practice, wheel another way, thus it was in the first and primitive commonwealths, and is yet in the integrity and cradle of well ordered polities: till corruption getteth ground; — ruder desires labouring after that which wiser considerations contemn; — every one having a liberty to amass and heap up riches, and they a licence or faculty to do or purchase anything.

§2. — This general and indifferent temper of mine doth more nearly dispose me to this noble virtue. It is a happiness to be born and framed unto virtue, and to grow up from the seeds of nature, rather than the inoculations and forced grafts of education: yet, if we are directed only by our particular natures, and regulate our inclinations by no higher rule than that of our reasons, we are but moralists; divinity will still call us heathens. Therefore this great work of charity must have other motives, ends, and impulsions. I give no alms to satisfy the hunger of my brother, but to fulfil and accomplish the will and command of my God; I draw not my purse for his sake that demands it, but his that enjoined it; I relieve no man upon the rhetorick of his miseries, nor to content mine own commiserating disposition; for this is still but moral charity, and an act that oweth more to passion than reason. He that relieves another upon the bare suggestion and bowels of pity doth not this so much for his sake as for his own; and so, by relieving them, we relieve ourselves also. It is as erroneous a conceit to redress other men's misfortunes upon the common considerations of merciful natures, that it may be one day our own case; for this is a sinister and politick kind of charity, whereby we seem to bespeak the pities of men in the like occasions. And truly I have observed that those professed eleemo-synaries, though in a crowd or multitude, do yet direct and place their petitions on a few and selected persons; there is surely a physiognomy, which those experienced and master mendicants observe, whereby they instantly discover a merciful aspect, and will single out a face, wherein they spy the signature and marks of mercy. For there are mystically in our faces certain characters which carry in them the motto of our souls, wherein he that can read A, B, C, may read our natures. I hold, moreover, that there is a phytognomy, or physiognomy, not only of men, but of plants and vegetables; and is every one of them some outward figures which hang as signs or bushes of their inward forms. The finger of

God hath left an inscription upon all his works, not graphical, or composed of letters, but of their several forms, constitutions, parts, and operations, which, aptly joined together, do make one word that doth express their natures. By these letters God calls the stars by their names; and by this alphabet Adam assigned to every creature a name peculiar to its nature. Now, there are, besides these characters in our faces, certain mystical figures in our hands, which I dare not call mere dashes, strokes *a la volee* or at random, because delineated by a pencil that never works in vain; and hereof I take more particular notice, because I carry that in mine own hand which I could never read of nor discover in another. Aristotle, I confess, in his acute and singular book of physiognomy, hath made no mention of chiromancy:[80] yet I believe the Egyptians, who were nearer addicted to those abstruse and mystical sciences, had a knowledge therein: to which those vagabond and counterfeit Egyptians did after[81] pretend, and perhaps retained a few corrupted principles, which sometimes might verify their prognosticks.

It is the common wonder of all men, how, among so many millions of faces, there should be none alike: now, contrary, I wonder as much how there should be any. He that shall consider how many thousand several words have been carelessly and without study composed out of twenty-four letters; withal, how many hundred lines there are to be drawn in the fabrick of one man; shall easily find that this variety is necessary: and it will be very hard that they shall so concur as to make one portrait like another. Let a painter carelessly limn out a million of faces, and you shall find them all different; yes, let him have his copy before him, yet, after all his art, there will remain a sensible distinction: for the pattern or example of everything is the perfectest in that kind, whereof we still come short, though we transcend or go beyond it; because herein it is wide, and agrees not in all points unto its copy. Nor doth the similitude of creatures disparage the variety of nature, nor any way confound the works of God. For even in things alike there is diversity; and those that do seem to accord do manifestly disagree. And thus is man like God; for, in the same things that we resemble him we are utterly different from him. There was never anything so like another as in all points to concur; there will ever some reserved difference slip in, to prevent the identity; without which two several things would not be alike, but the same, which is impossible.

§3. — But, to return from philosophy to charity, I hold not so narrow a conceit of this virtue as to conceive that to give alms is only to be charitable, or think a piece of liberality can comprehend the total of charity. Divinity hath wisely divided the act thereof into many branches, and hath taught us, in this narrow way, many paths unto goodness; as many ways as we may do good, so many ways we may be charitable. There are infirmities not only of body, but of soul and fortunes, which do require the merciful hand of our abilities. I cannot contemn a man for ignorance, but behold him with as much pity as I do Lazarus. It is no greater charity to clothe his body than apparel the nakedness of his soul. It is an honourable object to see the reasons of other men wear our liveries, and their borrowed understandings do homage to the bounty of ours. It is the cheapest way of beneficence, and, like the natural charity of the sun, illuminates another without obscuring itself. To be reserved and caitiff[82] in this part of goodness is the sordidest piece of covetousness, and more contemptible than the pecuniary avarice. To this (as calling myself a scholar) I am obliged by the duty of my condition. I make not therefore my head a grave, but a treasure of knowledge. I intend no monopoly, but a community in learning. I study not for my own sake only, but for theirs that study not for themselves. I envy no man that knows more than myself, but pity them that know less. I instruct no man as an exercise of my knowledge, or with an intent rather to nourish and keep it alive in mine own head than beget and propagate it in his. And, in the midst of all my endeavours, there is but one thought that dejects me, that my acquired parts must perish with myself, nor can be legacied among my honoured friends. I cannot fall out or contemn a man for an error, or conceive why a difference in opinion should divide an affection; for controversies, disputes, and argumentations, both in philosophy and in divinity, if they meet with discreet and peaceable natures, do not infringe the laws of charity. In all disputes, so much as there is of passion, so much there is of nothing to the purpose; for then reason, like a bad hound, spends upon a false scent, and forsakes the question first started. And this is one reason why controversies are never determined; for, though they be amply proposed, they are scarce at all handled; they do so swell with unnecessary digressions; and the parenthesis on the party is often as large as the main discourse upon the subject. The foundations of religion are already established, and the principles of salvation subscribed unto by all. There remain not many controversies worthy a passion, and yet never any dispute without, not only in divinity but inferior arts. What a [Greek omitted] and hot skirmish is betwixt S. and T. in Lucian![83] How do grammarians hack and slash for the genitive case in Jupiter![84] How do they break their own pates, to salve that of Priscian![85] "Si foret in terris, rideret Democritus." Yes, even amongst wiser militants, how many wounds have been given and credits slain, for the poor victory of an opinion, or beggarly conquest of a distinction! Scholars are men of peace, they bear no arms, but their tongues are sharper than Actius's razor.[86]

their pens carry farther, and give a louder report than thunder. I had rather stand the shock of a basilisko[87] than in the fury of a merciless pen. It is not mere zeal to learning, or devotion to the muses, that wiser princes patron the arts, and carry an indulgent aspect unto scholars; but a desire to have their names eternized by the memory of their writings, and a fear of the revengeful pen of succeeding ages: for these are the men that, when they have played their parts, and had their *exits*, must step out and give the moral of their scenes, and deliver unto posterity an inventory of their virtues and vices. And surely there goes a great deal of conscience to the compiling of an history: there is no reproach to the scandal of a story; it is such an authentick kind of falsehood, that with authority belies our good names to all nations and posterity.

§4. — There is another offence unto charity, which no author hath ever written of, and few take notice of, and that's the reproach, not of whole professions, mysteries, and conditions, but of whole nations, wherein by opprobrious epithets we miscall each other, and, by an uncharitable logick, from a disposition in a few, conclude a habit in all.

Le mutin Anglois, et le bravache Escossois Le bougre Italien, et le fol Francois; Le poltron Romain, le larron de Gascogne, L'Espagnol superbe, et l'Alleman yvrogue.

St Paul, that calls the Cretians liars, doth it but indirectly, and upon quotation of their own poet.[88] It is as bloody a thought in one way as Nero's was in another.[89] For by a word we wound a thousand, and at one blow assassin the honour of a nation. It is as complete a piece of madness to miscall and rave against the times; or think to recall men to reason by a fit of passion. Democritus, that thought to laugh the times into goodness, seems to me as deeply hypochondriack as Heraclitus, that bewailed them. It moves not my spleen to behold the multitude in their proper humours; that is, in their fits of folly and madness, as well understanding that wisdom is not profaned unto the world; and it is the privilege of a few to be virtuous. They that endeavour to abolish vice destroy also virtue; for contraries, though they destroy one another, are yet the life of one another. Thus virtue (abolish vice) is an idea. Again, the community of sin doth not disparage goodness; for, when vice gains upon the major part, virtue, in whom it remains, becomes more excellent, and, being lost in some, multiplies its goodness in others, which remain untouched, and persist entire in the general inundation. I can therefore behold vice without a satire, content only with an admonition, or instructive reprehension; for noble natures, and such as are capable of goodness, are railed into vice, that might as easily be admonished into virtue; and we should be all so far the orators of goodness as to protect her from the power of vice, and maintain the cause of injured truth. No man can justly censure or condemn another; because, indeed, no man truly knows another. This I perceive in myself; for I am in the dark to all the world, and my nearest friends behold me but in a cloud. Those that know me but superficially think less of me than I do of myself; those of my near acquaintance think more; God who truly knows me, knows that I am nothing: for he only beholds me, and all the world, who looks not on us through a derived ray, or a trajection of a sensible species, but beholds the substance without the help of accidents, and the forms of things, as we their operations. Further, no man can judge another, because no man knows himself; for we censure others but as they disagree from that humour which we fancy laudable in ourselves, and commend others but for that wherein they seem to quadrate and consent with us. So that in conclusion, all is but that we all condemn, self-love. 'Tis the general complaint of these times, and perhaps of those past, that charity grows cold; which I perceive most verified in those which do most manifest the fires and flames of zeal; for it is a virtue that best agrees with coldest natures, and such as are complexioned for humility. But how shall we expect charity towards others, when we are uncharitable to ourselves? "Charity begins at home," is the voice of the world; yet is every man his greatest enemy, and as it were his own executioner. "Non occides," is the commandment of God, yet scarce observed by any man; for I perceive every man is his own Atropos, and lends a hand to cut the thread of his own days. Cain was not therefore the first murderer, but Adam, who brought in death; whereof he beheld the practice and example in his own son Abel; and saw that verified in the experience of another which faith could not persuade him in the theory of himself.

§5. — There is, I think, no man that apprehends his own miseries less than myself; and no man that so nearly apprehends another's. I could lose an arm without a tear, and with few groans, methinks, be quartered into pieces; yet can I weep most seriously at a play, and receive with a true passion the counterfeit griefs of those known and professed impostures. It is a barbarous part of inhumanity to add unto any afflicted parties misery, or endeavour to multiply in any man a passion whose single nature is already above his patience. This was the greatest affliction of Job, and those oblique expostulations of his friends a deeper injury than the down-right blows of the devil. It is not the tears of our own eyes only, but of our friends also, that do exhaust the current of our sorrows; which, falling into many streams, runs more peaceably, and is contented with a narrower channel. It is an act within the power of charity, to translate a passion out of one breast into another, and to divide a sorrow almost out of itself; for an affliction, like a dimension, may be so divided as, if not indivisible, at least to become insensible. Now with my friend I desire not to share or participate, but to engross, his sorrows; that, by making them mine own, I may more easily discuss them: for in mine own reason, and within myself, I can command that which I cannot entreat without myself, and within the circle of another. I have often thought those noble pairs and examples of friendship, not so truly histories of what had been, as fictions of what should be; but I now perceive nothing in them but possibilities, nor anything in the heroick examples of Damon and Pythias, Achilles and Patroclus, which, methinks, upon some grounds, I could not perform within the narrow compass of myself. That a man should lay down his life for his friend seems strange to vulgar affections and such as confine themselves within that worldly principle, "Charity begins at home." For mine own part, I could never remember the relations that I held unto myself, nor the respect that I owe unto my own nature, in the cause of God, my country, and my friends. Next to these three, I do embrace myself. I confess I do not observe that order that the schools ordain our affections — to love our parents, wives, children, and then our friends; for, excepting the injunctions of religion, I do not find in myself such a necessary and indissoluble sympathy to all those of my blood. I hope I do not break the fifth commandment, if I conceive I may love my friend before the nearest of my blood, even those to whom I owe the principles of life. I never yet cast a true affection on a woman; but I have loved my friend, as I do virtue, my soul, my God. From hence, methinks, I do conceive how God loves man; what happiness there is in the love of God. Omitting all other, there are three most mystical unions; two natures in one person; three persons in one nature; one soul in two bodies. For though, indeed, they be really divided, yet are they so united, as they seem but one, and make rather a duality than two distinct souls.

§6. — There are wonders in true affection. It is a body of enigmas, mysteries, and riddles; wherein two so become one as they both become two: I love my friend before myself, and yet, methinks, I do not love him enough. Some few months hence, my multiplied affection will make me believe I have not loved him at all. When I am from him, I am dead till I be with him. United souls are not satisfied with embraces, but desire to be truly each other; which being impossible, these desires are infinite, and must proceed without a possibility of satisfaction. Another misery there is in affection; that whom we truly love like our own selves, we forget their looks, nor can our memory retain the idea of their faces: and it is no wonder, for they are ourselves, and our affection makes their looks our own. This noble affection falls not on vulgar and common constitutions; but on such as are marked for virtue. He that can love his friend with this noble ardour will in a competent degree effect all. Now, if we can bring our affections to look beyond the body, and cast an eye upon the soul, we have found out the true object, not only of friendship, but charity: and the greatest happiness that we can bequeath the soul is that wherein we all do place our last felicity, salvation; which, though it be not in our power to bestow, it is in our charity and pious invocations to desire, if not procure and further. I cannot contentedly frame a prayer for myself in particular, without a catalogue for my friends; nor request a happiness wherein my sociable disposition doth not desire the fellowship of my neighbour. I never hear the toll of a passing bell, though in my mirth, without my prayers and best wishes for the departing spirit. I cannot go to cure the body of my patient, but I forget my profession, and call unto God for his soul. I cannot see one say his prayers, but, instead of imitating him, I fall into supplication for him, who perhaps is no more to me than a common nature: and if God hath vouchsafed an ear to my supplications, there are surely many happy that never saw me, and enjoy the blessing of mine unknown devotions. To pray for enemies, that is, for their salvation, is no harsh precept, but the practice of our daily and ordinary devotions. I cannot believe the story of the Italian;[90] our bad wishes and uncharitable desires proceed no further than this life; it is the devil, and the uncharitable votes of hell, that desire our misery in the world to come.

§7. —"To do no injury nor take none" was a principle which, to my former years and impatient affections, seemed to contain enough of morality, but my more settled years, and Christian constitution, have fallen upon severer resolutions. I can hold there is no such things as injury; that if there be, there is no such injury as revenge, and no such revenge as the contempt of an injury: that to hate another is to malign himself; that the truest way to love another is to despise ourselves. I were unjust unto mine own conscience if I should say I am at variance with anything like myself. I find there are many pieces in this one fabrick of man; this frame is raised upon a mass of antipathies: I am one methinks but as the world, wherein notwithstanding there are a swarm of distinct essences, and in them another world of contrarieties; we carry private and domestick enemies within, public and more hostile adversaries without. The devil, that did but buffet St Paul, plays methinks at sharp[91] with me. Let me be nothing, if within the compass of myself, I do not find the battle of Lepanto,[92] passion against reason, reason against faith, faith against the devil, and my conscience against all. There is another man within me that's angry with me, rebukes, commands, and dastards me. I have no conscience of marble, to resist the hammer of more heavy offences: nor yet so soft and waxen, as to take the impression of each single peccadillo or scape of infirmity. I am of a strange belief, that it is as easy to be forgiven some sins as to commit some others. For my original sin, I hold it to be washed away in my baptism; for my actual transgressions, I compute and reckon with God but from my last repentance, sacrament, or general absolution; and therefore am not terrified with the sins or madness of my youth. I thank the goodness of God, I have no sins that want a name. I am not singular in offences; my transgressions are epidemical, and from the common breath of our corruption. For there are certain tempers of body which, matched with a humorous depravity of mind, do hath and produce vitiosities, whose newness and monstrosity of nature admits no name; this was the temper of that lecher that carnaled with a statua, and the constitution of Nero in his spintrian recreations. For the heavens are not only fruitful in new and unheard-of stars, the earth in plants and animals, but men's minds also in villany and vices. Now the dulness of my reason, and the vulgarity of my disposition, never prompted my invention nor solicited my affection unto any of these; — yet even those common and quotidian infirmities that so necessarily attend me, and do seem to be my very nature, have so dejected me, so broken the estimation that I should have otherwise of myself, that I repute myself the most abject piece of mortality. Divines prescribe a fit of sorrow to repentance: there goes indignation, anger, sorrow, hatred, into mine, passions of a con trary nature, which neither seem to suit with this action, nor my proper constitution. It is no breach of charity to ourselves to be at variance with our vices, nor to abhor that part of us, which is an enemy to the ground of charity, our God; wherein we do but imitate our great selves, the world, whose divided antipathies and contrary faces do yet carry a charitable regard unto the whole, by their particular discords preserving the common harmony, and keeping in fetters those powers, whose rebellions, once masters, might be the ruin of all.

§8. — I thank God, amongst those millions of vices I do inherit and hold from Adam, I have escaped one, and that a mortal enemy to charity — the first and father sin, not only of man, but of the devil — pride; a vice whose name is comprehended in a monosyllable, but in its nature not circumscribed with a world, I have escaped it in a condition that can hardly avoid it. Those petty acquisitions and reputed perfections, that advance and elevate the conceits of other men, add no feathers unto mine. I have seen a grammarian tower and plume himself over a single line in Horace, and show more pride, in the construction of one ode, than the author in the composure of the whole book. For my own part, besides the jargon and *patois* of several provinces, I understand no less than six languages; yet I protest I have no higher conceit of myself than had our fathers before the confusion of Babel, when there was but one language in the world, and none to boast himself either linguist or critick. I have not only seen several countries, beheld the nature of their climes, the chorography of their provinces, topography of their cities, but understood their several laws, customs, and policies; yet cannot all this persuade the dulness of my spirit unto such an opinion of myself as I behold in nimbler and conceited heads, that never looked a degree beyond their nests. I know the names and somewhat more of all the constellations in my horizon; yet I have seen a prating mariner, that could only name the pointers and the north-star, out-talk me, and conceit himself a whole sphere above me. I know most of the plants of my country, and of those about me, yet methinks I do not know so many as when I did but know a hundred, and had scarcely ever simpled further than Cheapside. For, indeed, heads of capacity, and such as are not full with a handful or easy measure of knowledge, think they know nothing till they know all; which being impossible, they fall upon the opinion of Socrates, and only know they know not anything. I cannot think that Homer pined away upon the riddle of the fishermen, or that Aristotle, who understood the uncertainty of knowledge, and confessed so often the reason of man too weak for the works of nature, did ever drown himself upon the flux and reflux of Euripus.[23] We do but learn, today, what our better advanced judgments will unteach tomorrow; and Aristotle doth but instruct us, as Plato did him, that is, to confute himself. I have run through all sorts, yet find no rest in any: though our first studies and junior endeavours may style us Peripateticks, Stoicks, or Academicks, yet I perceive the wisest heads prove, at last, almost all Scepticks,[24] and stand like Janus in the field of knowledge. I have therefore one common and authentick philosophy I learned in the schools, whereby I discourse and satisfy the reason of other men; another more reserved, and drawn from experience, whereby I content mine own. Solomon, that complained of ignorance in the height of knowledge, hath not only humbled my conceits, but discouraged my endeavours. There is yet another conceit that hath sometimes made me shut my books, which tells me it is a vanity to waste our days in the blind pursuit of knowledge: it is but attending a little longer, and we shall enjoy that, by instinct and infusion, which we endeavour at here by labour and inquisition. It is better to sit down in a modest ignorance, and rest contented with the natural blessing of our own reasons, than by the uncertain knowledge of this life with sweat and vexation, which death gives every fool gratis, and is an accessary of our glorification.

§9. — I was never yet once, and commend their resolutions who never marry twice. Not that I disallow of second marriage; as neither in all cases of polygamy, which considering some times, and the unequal number of both sexes, may be also necessary. The whole world was made for man, but the twelfth part of man for woman. Man is the whole world, and the breath of God; woman the rib and crooked piece of man. I could be content that we might procreate like trees, without conjunction, or that there were any way to perpetuate the world without this trivial and vulgar way of coition: it is the foolishest act a wise man commits in all his life, nor is there anything that will more deject his cooled imagination, when he shall consider what an odd and unworthy piece of folly he hath committed. I speak not in prejudice, nor am averse from that sweet sex, but naturally amorous of all that is beautiful. I can look a whole day with delight upon a handsome picture, though it be but of an horse. It is my temper, and I like it the better, to affect all harmony; and sure there is musick, even in the beauty and the silent note which Cupid strikes, far sweeter than the sound of an instrument. For there is a musick wherever there is a harmony, order, or proportion; and thus far we may maintain "the musick of the spheres:" for those well-ordered motions, and regular paces, though they give no sound unto the ear, yet to the understanding they strike a note most full of harmony. Whatsoever is harmonically composed delights in harmony, which makes me much distrust the symmetry of those heads which declaim against all church-musick. For myself, not only from my obedience but my particular genius I do embrace it: for even that vulgar and tavern-musick which makes one man merry, another mad, strikes in me a deep fit of devotion, and a profound contemplation of the first composer. There is something in it of divinity more than the ear discovers: it is an hieroglyphical and shadowed lesson of the whole world, and creatures of God — such a melody to the ear, as the whole world, well understood, would afford the understanding. In brief, it is a sensible fit of that harmony which intellectually sounds in the ears of God. I will not say, with Plato, the soul is an harmony, but harmonical, and hath its nearest sympathy unto musick: thus some, whose temper of body agrees, and humours the constitution of * "Urbem a Romam in principio reges habuere." their souls, are born poets, though indeed all are naturally inclined unto rhythm. This made Tacitus, in the very first line of his story, fall upon a verse;* and Cicero, the worst of poets, but declaiming for a poet, falls in the very first sentence upon a * "In qua me non inferior mediocriter esse."— *Pro Archia Poeta.* perfect hexameter.* I feel not in me those sordid and unchristian desires of my profession; I do not secretly implore and wish for plagues, rejoice at famines, revolve ephemerides and almanacks in expectation of malignant aspects, fatal conjunctions, and eclipses. I rejoice not at unwholesome springs nor unseasonable winters: my prayer goes with the husbandman's; I desire everything in its proper season, that neither men nor the times be out of temper. Let me be sick myself, if sometimes the malady of my patient be not a disease unto me. I desire rather to cure his infirmities than my own necessities. Where I do him no good, methinks it is scarce honest gain, though I confess 'tis but the worthy salary of our well intended endeavours. I am not only ashamed but heartily sorry, that, besides death, there are diseases incurable; yet not for my own sake or that they be beyond my art, but for the general cause and sake of humanity, whose common cause I apprehend as mine own. And, to speak more generally, those three noble professions which all civil commonwealths do honour, are raised upon the fall of Adam, and are not any way exempt from their infirmities. There are not only diseases incurable in physick, but cases indissolvable in law, vices incorrigible in divinity. If general councils may err, I do not see why particular courts should be infallible: their perfectest rules are raised upon the erroneous reasons of man, and the laws of one do but condemn the rules of another; as Aristotle oft-times the opinions of his predecessors, because, though agreeable to reason, yet were not consonant to his own rules and the logick of his proper principles. Again — to speak nothing of the sin against the Holy Ghost, whose cure not only, but whose nature is unknown — I can cure the gout or stone in some, sooner than divinity, pride, or avarice in others. I can cure vices by physick when they remain incurable by divinity, and they shall obey my pills when they contemn their precepts. I boast nothing, but plainly say, we all labour against our own cure; for death is the cure of all diseases. There is no *catholicon* or universal remedy I know, but this, which though nauseous to queasy stomachs, yet to prepared appetites is nectar, and a pleasant potion of im mortality.

§10. — For my conversation, it is, like the sun's, with all men, and with a friendly aspect to good and bad. Methinks there is no man bad; and the worst best, that is, while they are kept within the circle of those qualities wherein they are good. There is no man's mind of so discordant and jarring a temper, to which a tuneable disposition may not strike a harmony. *Magnae virtutes, nec minora vitia;* it is the posy[95] of the best natures, and may be inverted on the worst. There are, in the most depraved and venomous dispositions, certain pieces that remain untouched, which by an *antiperistasis*[96] become more excellent, or by the excellency of their antipathies are able to preserve themselves from the contagion of their enemy vices, and persist entire beyond the general corruption. For it is also thus in nature: the greatest balsams do lie enveloped in the bodies of the most powerful corrosives. I say moreover, and I ground upon experience, that poisons contain within themselves their own antidote, and that which preserves them from the venom of themselves; without which they were not deleterious to others only, but to themselves also. But it is the corruption that I fear within me; not the contagion of commerce without me. 'Tis that unruly regiment within me, that will destroy me; 'tis that I do infect myself; the man without a navel[97] yet lives in me. I feel that original canker corrode and devour me: and therefore, "Defenda me, Dios, de me!" "Lord, deliver me from myself!" is a part of my litany, and the first voice of my retired imaginations. There is no man alone, because every man is a * "Cic. de Off.," I. iii. microcosm, and carries the whole world about him. "Nunquam minus solus quam cum solus,"* though it be the apothegm of a wise man is yet true in the mouth of a fool: for indeed, though in a wilderness, a man is never alone; not only because he is with himself, and his own thoughts, but because he is with the devil, who ever consorts with our solitude, and is that unruly rebel that musters up those disordered motions which accompany our sequestered imaginations. And to speak more narrowly, there is no such thing as solitude, nor anything that can be said to be alone, and by itself, but God; — who is his own circle, and can subsist by himself; all others, besides their dissimilary and heterogeneous parts, which in a manner multiply their natures, cannot subsist without the concourse of God, and the society of that hand which doth uphold their natures. In brief, there can be nothing truly alone, and by its self, which is not truly one, and such is only God: all others do transcend an unity, and so by consequence are many.

§11. — Now for my life, it is a miracle of thirty years, which to relate, were not a history, but a piece of poetry, and would sound to common ears like a fable. For the world, I count it not an inn, but an hospital; and a place not to live, but to die in. The world that I regard is myself; it is the microcosm of my own frame that I cast mine eye on: for the other, I use it but like my globe, and turn it round sometimes for my recreation. Men that look upon my outside, perusing only my condition and fortunes, do err in my altitude; for I am above Atlas's shoulders.[98] The earth is a point not only in respect of the heavens above us, but of the heavenly and celestial part within us. That mass of flesh that circumscribes me limits not my mind. That surface that tells the heavens it hath an end cannot persuade me I have any. I take my circle to be above three hundred and sixty. Though the number of the ark do measure my body, it comprehendeth not my mind. Whilst I study to find how I am a microcosm, or little world, I find myself something more than the great. There is surely a piece of divinity in us; something that was before the elements, and owes no homage unto the sun. Nature tells me, I am the image of God, as well as Scripture. He that understands not thus much hath not his introduction or first lesson, and is yet to begin the alphabet of man. Let me not injure the felicity of others, if I say I am as happy as any. *Ruat coelum, fiat voluntas tua,*" salveth all; so that, whatsoever happens, it is but what our daily prayers desire. In brief, I am content; and what should providence add more? Surely this is it we call happiness, and this do I enjoy; with this I am happy in a dream, and as content to enjoy a happiness in a fancy, as others in a more apparent truth and reality. There is surely a nearer apprehension of anything that delights us, in our dreams, than in our waked senses. Without this I were unhappy; for my awaked judgment discontents me, ever whispering unto me that I am from my friend, but my friendly dreams in the night requite me, and make me think I am within his arms. I thank God for my happy dreams, as I do for my good rest; for there is a satisfaction in them unto reasonable desires, and such as can be content with a fit of happiness. And surely it is not a melancholy conceit to think we are all asleep in this world, and that the conceits of this life are as mere dreams, to those of the next, as the phantasms of the night, to the conceits of the day. There is an equal delusion in both; and the one doth but seem to be the emblem or picture of the other. We are somewhat more than ourselves in our sleeps; and the slumber of the body seems to be but the waking of the soul. It is the ligation of sense, but the liberty of reason; and our waking conceptions do not match the fancies of our sleeps. At my nativity, my ascendant was the watery sign of *Scorpio*. I was born in the planetary hour of *Saturn*, and I think I have a piece of that leaden planet in me. I am no way facetious, nor disposed for the mirth and galliardise[99] of company; yet in one dream I can compose a whole comedy, behold the action, apprehend the jests, and laugh myself awake at the con ceits thereof. Were my memory as faithful as my reason is then fruitful, I would never study but in my dreams, and this time also would I choose for my devotions: but our grosser memories have then so little hold of our abstracted understandings, that they forget the story, and can only relate to our awaked souls a confused and broken tale of that which hath passed. Aristotle, who hath written a singular tract of sleep, hath not, methinks, thoroughly defined it; nor yet Galen, though he seem to have corrected it; for those *noctambulos* and night-walkers, though in their sleep, do yet enjoy the action of their senses. We must therefore say that there is something in us that is not in the jurisdiction of Morpheus; and that those abstracted and ecstatick souls do walk about in their own corpses, as spirits with the bodies they assume, wherein they seem to hear, see, and feel, though indeed the organs are destitute of sense, and their natures of those faculties that should inform them. Thus it is observed, that men sometimes, upon the hour of their departure, do speak and reason above themselves. For then the soul beginning to be freed from the ligaments of the body, begins to reason like herself, and to discourse in a strain above mortality.

§12. — We term sleep a death; and yet it is waking that kills us, and destroys those spirits that are the house of life. 'Tis indeed a part of life that best expresseth death; for every man truly lives, so long as he acts his nature, or some way makes good the faculties of himself. Themistocles therefore, that slew his soldier in his sleep, was a merciful executioner: 'tis a kind of punishment the mildness of no laws hath invented; I wonder the fancy of Lucan and Seneca did not discover it. It is that death by which we may be literally said to die daily; a death which Adam died before his mortality; a death whereby we live a middle and moderating point between life and death. In fine, so like death, I dare not trust it without my prayers, and an half adieu unto the world, and take my farewell in a colloquy with God:—

The night is come, like to the day; Depart not thou, great God, away. Let not my sins, black as the night, Eclipse the lustre of thy light. Keep still in my horizon; for to me The sun makes not the day, but thee. Thou whose nature cannot sleep, On my temples sentry keep; Guard me 'gainst those watchful foes, Whose eyes are open while mine close. Let no dreams my head infest, But such as Jacob's temples blest. While I do rest, my soul advance: Make my sleep a holy trance: That I may, my rest being wrought, Awake into some holy thought, And with as active vigour run My course as doth the nimble sun. Sleep is a death; — Oh make me try, By sleeping, what it is to die! And as gently lay my head On my grave, as now my bed. Howe'er I rest, great God, let me Awake again at last with thee. And thus assured, behold I lie Securely, or to wake or die. These are my drowsy days; in vain I do now wake to sleep again: Oh come that hour, when I shall never Sleep again, but wake for ever!

This is the dormitive I take to bedward; I need no other *laudanum* than this to make me sleep; after which I close mine eyes in security, content to take my leave of the sun, and sleep unto the resurrection.

§13. — The method I should use in distributive justice, I often observe in commutative; and keep a geometrical proportion in both, whereby becoming equable to others, I become unjust to myself, and supererogate in that common principle, "Do unto others as thou wouldst be done unto thyself." I was not born unto riches, neither is it, I think, my star to be wealthy; or if it were, the freedom of my mind, and frankness of my disposition, were able to contradict and cross my fates: for to me avarice seems not so much a vice, as a deplorable piece of madness; to conceive ourselves urinals, or be persuaded that we are dead, is not so ridiculous, nor so many degrees beyond the power of hellebore,[100] as this. The opinions of theory, and positions of men, are not so void of reason, as their practised conclusions. Some have held that snow is black, that the earth moves, that the soul is air, fire, water; but all this is philosophy: and there is no delirium, if we do but speculate the folly and indisputable dotage of avarice. To that subterraneous idol, and god of the earth, I do confess I am an atheist. I cannot persuade myself to honour that the world adores; whatsoever virtue its prepared substance may have within my body, it hath no influence nor operation without. I would not entertain a base design, or an action that should call me villain, for the Indies; and for this only do I love and honour my own soul, and have methinks two arms too few to embrace myself. Aristotle is too severe, that will not allow us to be truly liberal without wealth, and the bountiful hand of fortune; if this be true, I must confess I am charitable only in my liberal intentions, and bountiful well wishes. But if the example of the mite be not only an act of wonder, but an example of the noblest charity, surely poor men may also build hospitals, and the rich alone have not erected cathedrals. I have a private method which others observe not; I take the opportunity of myself to do good; I borrow occasion of charity from my own necessities, and supply the wants of others, when I am in most need myself: for it is an honest stratagem to take advantage of ourselves, and so to husband the acts of virtue, that, where they are defective in one circumstance, they may repay their want, and multiply their goodness in another. I have not Peru in my desires, but a competence and ability to perform those good works to which he hath inclined my nature. He is rich who hath enough to be charitable; and it is hard to be so poor that a noble mind may not find a way to this piece of goodness. "He that giveth to the poor lendeth to the Lord:" there is more rhetorick in that one sentence than in a library of sermons. And indeed, if those sentences were understood by the reader with the same emphasis as they are delivered by the author, we needed not those volumes of instructions, but might be honest by an epitome. Upon this motive only I cannot behold a beggar without relieving his necessities with my purse, or his soul with my prayers. These scenical and accidental differences between us cannot make me forget that common and untoucht part of us both: there is under these centoes[101] and miserable outsides, those mutilate and semi bodies, a soul of the same alloy with our own, whose genealogy is God's as well as ours, and * "The poor ye have always with you." in as fair a way to salvation as ourselves. Statists that labour to contrive a commonwealth without our poverty take away the object of charity; not understanding only the commonwealth of a Christian, but forgetting the prophecy of Christ.*

§14. — Now, there is another part of charity, which is the basis and pillar of this, and that is the love of God, for whom we love our neighbour; for this I think charity, to love God for himself, and our neighbour for God. And all that is truly amiable is God, or as it were a divided piece of him, that retains a reflex or shadow of himself. Nor is it strange that we should place affection on that which is invisible: all that we truly love is thus. What we adore under affection of our senses deserves not the honour of so pure a title. Thus we adore virtue, though to the eyes of sense she be invisible. Thus that part of our noble friends that we love is not that part that we embrace, but that insensible part that our arms cannot embrace. God being all goodness, can love nothing but himself; he loves us but for that part which is as it were himself, and the traduction of his Holy Spirit. Let us call to assize the loves of our parents, the affection of our wives and children, and they are all dumb shows and dreams, without reality, truth, or constancy. For first there is a strong bond of affection between us and our parents; yet how easily dissolved! We betake ourselves to a woman, forgetting our mother in a wife, and the womb that bare us in that which shall bear our image. This woman blessing us with children, our affection leaves the level it held before, and sinks from our bed unto our issue and picture of posterity: where affection holds no steady mansion; they growing up in years, desire our ends; or, applying themselves to a woman, take a lawful way to love another better than ourselves. Thus I perceive a man may be buried alive, and behold his grave in his own issue.

§15. — I conclude therefore, and say, there is no * Who holds that the sun is the centre of the world. happiness under (or, as Copernicus* will have it, above) the sun; nor any crambe[102] in that repeated verity and burthen of all the wisdom of Solomon: "All is vanity and vexation of spirit;" there is no felicity in that the world adores. Aristotle, whilst he labours to refute the *ideas* of Plato, falls upon one himself: for his *summum bonum* is a chimaera; and there is no such thing as his felicity. That wherein God himself is happy, the holy angels are happy, in whose defect the devils are unhappy; — that dare I call happiness: whatsoever conduceth unto this, may, with an easy metaphor, deserve that name; whatsoever else the world terms happiness is, to me, a story out of Pliny, a tale of Bocace or

Malizspini, an apparition or neat delusion, wherein there is no more of happiness than the name. Bless me in this life with but the peace of my conscience, command of my affections, the love of thyself and my dearest friends, and I shall be happy enough to pity Caesar! These are, O Lord, the humble desires of my most reasonable ambition, and all I dare call happiness on earth; wherein I set no rule or limit to thy hand or providence; dispose of me according to the wisdom of thy pleasure. Thy will be done, though in my own undoing.

79. From the Spanish "Dorado," a gilt head.

80. Sir T. Browne treats of chiromancy, or the art of telling fortunes by means of lines in the hands, in his "Vulgar Errors," lib. v. cap. 23.

81. Gypsies.

82. S. Wilkin says that here this word means niggardly.

83. In the dialogue, "judicium vocalium," the vowels are the judges, and [Greek Sigma omitted] complains that T has deprived him of many letters that ought to begin with [Greek Sigma omitted].

84. If Jovis or Jupitris.

85. The celebrated Roman grammarian. A proverbial phrase for the violation of grammar was "Breaking Priscian's head."

86. Livy says, Actius Nevius cut a whetstone through with a razor.

87. A kind of lizard that was supposed to kill all it looked at —

"Whose baneful eye

Wounds at a glance, so that the soundest dye."

— *De Bartas*, 6me jour 1me sem.

88. Epimenides (Titus x. 12)—

[Greek omitted]

89. Nero having heard a person say, "When I am dead, let earth be mingled with fire," replied, "Yes, while I live."— Suetonius, *Vit. Nero.*

90. Alluding to the story of the Italian, who, having been provoked by a person he met, put a poniard to his heart, and threatened to kill him if he would not blaspheme God; and the stranger doing so, the Italian killed him at once, that he might be damned, having no time to repent.

91. A rapier or small sword.

92. The battle here referred to was the one between Don John of Austria and the Turkish fleet, near Lepanto, in 1571. The battle of Lepanto (that is, the capture of the town by the Turks) did not take place till 1678.

93. Several authors say that Aristotle died of grief because he could not find out the reason for the ebb and flow of the tide in Epirus.

94. Who deny that there is such a thing as science.

95. A motto on a ring or cup. In an old will, 1655, there is this passage: "I give a cup of silver gilt to have this posy written in the margin:—

"When the drink is out, and the bottom you may see,

Remember your brother I. G."

96. The opposition of a contrary quality, by which the quality it opposes becomes heightened.

97. Adam as he was created and not born.

98. Meaning a world, as Atlas supported the world on his shoulders.

99. Merriment. Johnson says that this is the only place where the word is found.

100. Said to be a cure for madness.

101. Patched garments.

[102]. A game. A kind of capping verses, in which, if any one repeated what had been said before, he paid a forfeit.

Made in the USA
Las Vegas, NV
23 September 2021